QuickSCID-5

T0200321

QUICK STRUCTURED CLINICAL INTERVIEW FOR DSM-5® DISORDERS

Michael B. First, M.D.
Professor of Clinical Psychiatry, Columbia University, and Research Psychiatrist,
Division of Behavioral Health Services and Policy Research and Diagnosis and Assessment Lab,
New York State Psychiatric Institute,
New York, New York

Janet B. W. Williams, Ph.D.
Professor Emerita of Clinical Psychiatric Social Work (in Psychiatry and Neurology),
Columbia University, and Research Scientist and Deputy Chief, Biometrics Research Department (Retired),
New York State Psychiatric Institute, New York, New York;
Senior Vice President of Global Science (Retired), MedAvante Inc., Hamilton, New Jersey

Purchase includes a Limited Photocopy License. Customers may make up to 200 copies of the assessments for private clinical use without permission.

Subject/Patient: _____

Date of Interview: _____ _____ _____
　　　　　　　　　　　month　day　year

Clinician: _____

Note: The authors have worked to ensure that all information in this book is accurate at the time of publication and consistent with general psychiatric and medical standards, and that information concerning drug dosages, schedules, and routes of administration is accurate at the time of publication and consistent with standards set by the U.S. Food and Drug Administration and the general medical community. As medical research and practice continue to advance, however, therapeutic standards may change. Moreover, specific situations may require a specific therapeutic response not included in this book. For these reasons and because human and mechanical errors sometimes occur, we recommend that readers follow the advice of physicians directly involved in their care or the care of a member of their family.

Books published by American Psychiatric Association Publishing represent the findings, conclusions, and views of the individual authors and do not necessarily represent the policies and opinions of American Psychiatric Association Publishing or the American Psychiatric Association.

If you wish to buy 50 or more copies of the same title, please go to www.appi.org/specialdiscounts for more information.

Copyright © 2021 Michael B. First and Janet B.W. Williams
ALL RIGHTS RESERVED

DSM and DSM-5 are registered trademarks of the American Psychiatric Association. Use of these terms is prohibited without permission of the American Psychiatric Association.

DSM-5® diagnostic criteria are reprinted or adapted with permission from American Psychiatric Association: *Diagnostic and Statistical Manual of Mental Disorders,* Fifth Edition. Arlington VA, American Psychiatric Association, 2013. Copyright © 2013 American Psychiatric Association. Used with permission.

Unless authorized in writing by the American Psychiatric Association (APA), no part of the DSM-5® criteria may be reproduced or used in a manner inconsistent with the APA's copyright. This prohibition applies to unauthorized uses or reproductions in any form, including electronic applications. Correspondence regarding copyright permission for DSM-5 criteria should be directed to DSM Permissions, American Psychiatric Association Publishing, 800 Maine Ave. SW, Suite 900, Washington, DC 20024-2812.

No part of the QuickSCID-5 may be photocopied, reproduced, stored in a retrieval system, or transmitted, in any form or by any means, without obtaining permission in writing from American Psychiatric Association Publishing, or as expressly permitted by law, by license, or by terms agreed with the appropriate reproduction rights organization. All such inquiries, including those concerning reproduction outside the scope of the above, should be sent to Rights Department, American Psychiatric Association Publishing, 800 Maine Ave. SW, Suite 900, Washington, DC 20024-2812 or via the online permissions form located at: http://www.appi.org/permissions. For more information, please visit the SCID products page on www.appi.org.

For citation: First MB, Williams JBW: Quick Structured Clinical Interview for DSM-5® Disorders (QuickSCID-5). Washington, DC, American Psychiatric Association, 2021

Manufactured in the United States of America on acid-free paper
24 23 22 21 20   5 4 3 2 1

American Psychiatric Association Publishing
800 Maine Ave. SW
Suite 900
Washington, DC 20024-2812
www.appi.org

Limited Photocopy License

Purchase includes a license to photocopy QuickSCID-5 interview components for private clinical assessment use, up to 200 total copies per customer without charge. Outside of the Limited Photocopy License, the QuickSCID-5 may not be reproduced, stored in a retrieval system, or transmitted, in any form or by any means, without obtaining permission in writing from American Psychiatric Association Publishing, or as expressly permitted by law, by license, or by terms agreed with the appropriate reproduction rights organization.

Contents

Acknowledgments

The authors gratefully acknowledge the following individuals who provided helpful comments on drafts of the QuickSCID:

- Madeline M. Alexander
- Bernadette D'Souza
- Nina Engelhardt
- Angela Kirby
- Ari Lowell

QuickSCID-5 Diagnostic Summary

Check if present	Diagnoses	Item number and page number where diagnosis is made
	Bipolar I Disorder (lifetime) ____ Currently Manic (**A34**, Page A-7) ____ Currently Depressed (**A10**, Page A-2)	**A70** (Page A-15)
	Bipolar II Disorder (lifetime) ____ Currently Hypomanic (**A45**, Page A-9) ____ Currently Depressed (**A10**, Page A-2)	**A71** (Page A-15)
	Other Specified Bipolar Disorder	**A72** (Page A-15)
	Major Depressive Disorder ____ Currently in an episode (**A10**, Page A-2)	**A73** (Page A-15)
	Other Specified Depressive Disorder	**A74** (Page A-15)
	Possible Lifetime Psychotic Disorder	**B13** (Page B-3)
	Possible Current Psychotic Disorder	**B14** (Page B-3)
	Alcohol Use Disorder (past year) ____ Mild ____ Moderate ____ Severe	**C13** (Page C-3)
	Nonalcohol Substance Use Disorder (past year) *Name of specific substance:* _____ ____ Mild ____ Moderate ____ Severe	**C35** (Page C-7)
	Panic Disorder (current)	**D16** (Page D-2)
	Agoraphobia (current)	**D22** (Page D-3)
	Social Anxiety Disorder (current)	**D28** (Page D-4)
	Generalized Anxiety Disorder (current)	**D37** (Page D-6)
	Obsessive-Compulsive Disorder (current)	**E5** (Page E-2)
	Attention-Deficit/Hyperactivity Disorder (current)	**F24** (Page F-4)
	Posttraumatic Stress Disorder (current)	**G18** (Page G-3)
	Anorexia Nervosa (current)	**H3** (Page H-1)
	Bulimia Nervosa (current)	**H7** (Page H-2)
	Binge-Eating Disorder (current)	**H14** (Page H-3)
	Possible Other Disorders: _____	**I1-I14** (Pages I-1 to I-3)

Check if present	Diagnoses	Item number and page number where diagnosis is made
	Probable Mental Disorder due to Another Medical Condition Medical condition: _____ Indicate type of mental disorder: __ Depressive Disorder __ Bipolar and Related Disorder __ Anxiety Disorder __ Obsessive-Compulsive and Related Disorder	**J1** (Page J-1)
	Probable Substance/Medication-Induced Mental Disorder Substance/medication: _____ Indicate type of mental disorder: __ Depressive Disorder __ Bipolar and Related Disorder __ Anxiety Disorder __ Obsessive-Compulsive and Related Disorder	**J2** (Page J-1)

QuickSCID-5 Instructions

QuickSCID-5 is a fully structured interview adapted from the *Structured Clinical Interview for DSM-5 Disorders (SCID-5)*; it is designed to be much quicker to administer. QuickSCID-5 consists of 10 free-standing modules: Module A (Mood Episodes and Disorders), Module B (Psychotic Symptom Screen), Module C (Alcohol and Other Substance Use Disorders), Module D (Anxiety Disorders), Module E (Obsessive-Compulsive Disorder); Module F (Attention-Deficit/Hyperactivity Disorder), Module G (Posttraumatic Stress Disorder), Module H (Eating Disorders), Module I (Screening for Other Disorders), and Module J (Rule Out Mental Disorder due to Another Medical Condition and/or Substance/Medication-Induced Disorders). With this modular design, only modules of interest need to be administered. The QuickSCID-5 begins with an optional overview that asks about current symptoms and past treatment and includes an assessment of current and past suicidal ideation and behavior. The overview can be skipped if the information assessed in this section (i.e., demographics, history of current illness, past psychiatric history, medical problems, suicidal ideation/behavior) is already known to the interviewer.

Diagnostic Items and Item Codes

The QuickSCID-5 consists of a series of "diagnostic items" that correspond to the elements that compose the individual DSM-5 diagnoses (e.g., criteria, algorithmic rules). The interviewer rates each diagnostic item sequentially unless instructed to skip ahead, usually when the disorder being evaluated is ruled out. Each diagnostic item is uniquely identified by an item code in bold typeface, consisting of a letter that refers to the module being evaluated and a number (e.g., **A2**), which is placed along the left and right sides of the diagnostic item. Page numbers consist of a letter indicating the module, followed by a hyphen and a number (e.g., **page A-5**).

The item codes in the QuickSCID-5 serve three purposes:

- to indicate the destination item within skip instructions (e.g., "skip to **A12** (*Past Major Depressive Episode*), **page A-3**").
- to indicate which items should be counted toward meeting the diagnostic threshold within instructions that require counting the number of "+" ratings (e.g., *"If fewer than five items (A1–A9) are coded '+,' skip to **A12** (Past Major Depressive Episode), **page A-3**. Otherwise, continue with **A10**."*).
- to provide standardized designations for data items for later analysis.

Rating Diagnostic Items

The interviewer reads each question to the subject/patient and rates the diagnostic item as either "+" or "−," depending on the subject/patient's answer. In most cases, a "+" rating is given if <u>any</u> of the questions within the single item are answered "yes" by the subject/patient. For example, diagnostic item **A7**, which assesses DSM-5 criterion A.7 for Major Depressive Episode (feelings of worthlessness or excessive or inappropriate guilt), includes two interview questions. The diagnostic item is rated "+" if <u>either</u> (or both) question is answered "yes" or rated "−" only if <u>both</u> questions are answered "no." It is recommended that the interviewer ask the subject/patient to provide examples for "yes" answers, especially if there is any uncertainty as to whether the subject/patient may have misunderstood the question. In general, asking the subject/patient to provide descriptive examples will reduce the potential for false positive diagnoses.

A7	**In the past 2 weeks, have you been feeling worthless nearly every day?** **What about feeling guilty about things you have done or not done, nearly every day (not including feeling guilty about not taking care of things because you have been sick)?**	− +	A7

In a few cases, a "+" rating is given only if <u>both</u> questions are answered "yes," a requirement that is indicated by an instruction to "Code '+' only if 'YES' to both elevated mood and increased energy." (See example below.)

A23	**Over the past few days, have you been feeling so good, "high," excited, or "on top of the world" that other people thought you were not your normal self? Was that more than just feeling good?** IF YES: **Have you also felt like you were "hyper" or "wired" and had an unusual amount of energy or that you were much more active than is typical for you?** *Note: Code "+" only if "YES" to both elevated mood and increased energy.*	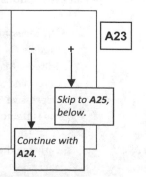	A23

QuickSCID-5 Conventions

- Interview questions to be read verbatim are printed in **bold** typeface.

- Instructions and explanatory notes to the interviewer are in unbolded *italics*.

- Many of the QuickSCID-5 questions contain unbolded phrases in all caps that are enclosed in parentheses, such as "(5% OF PERSON'S BODY WEIGHT)," "(FEARED SOCIAL OR PERFORMANCE SITUATION[S])," and "(SXS RATED '+')," and so forth. Rather than reading these verbatim, the interviewer, by convention, inserts subject/patient-specific words in place of these designations. So the parenthetical phrase "5% OF PERSON'S BODY WEIGHT" would be replaced by the interviewer's estimate of what 5% of the subject/patient's body weight would be; "FEARED SOCIAL OR PERFORMANCE SITUATIONS" would be replaced by the particular social or performance situations that the subject/patient fears and avoids; and "SXS RATED '+'" which appears in the assessment of ADHD, would be replaced by a recounting of those ADHD symptoms that had been coded "+."

- Most DSM-5 disorders require symptoms to be present during and within a particular time frame (e.g., 12 months for Substance Use Disorder). The applicability of a particular time frame to the set of questions that follow it is indicated by an initial statement that ends in an ellipsis, such as "During the past 12 months ..." Questions assessing the syndromal symptoms that apply to that time frame are indicated by a corresponding ellipsis preceding the question. For example, the assessment of Alcohol Use Disorder begins with "During the past 12 months ...," and the first question is "... have you found that once you started drinking you ended up drinking much more than you intended to?" The interviewer should therefore begin each question with the applicable time frame, e.g., "During the past 12 months, have you found that once you started drinking ...?" Studies of memory and recall demonstrate that subjects/patients are more accurate in their recounting of events if questions are anchored to specific date ranges as opposed to time intervals. For this reason, questions inquiring about the presence of a symptom during a particular time interval (e.g., "During the past 6 months ...") have been augmented by the phrase "since (SIX MONTHS AGO)," which requires the interviewer to use both the time interval and the exact date range in the question. For example, in the determination of whether symptoms of Agoraphobia have been present during the past 6 months, the initial question is "In the past 6 months, since (6 MONTHS AGO), have you been very anxious about or afraid of a number of different situations like going out of the house alone, being in crowds, going to stores, standing in lines, or traveling on buses or trains?" When reading this question to the subject/patient in the context of an interview administered in the middle of December, the interviewer would ask "During the past 6 months, since this past July, have you been very anxious about or afraid of a number of different situations like ...?"

Ruling Out Medical Conditions and Substances or Medications as Etiological Factors

After making the diagnosis of certain disorders or symptoms (i.e., Major Depressive Episode, Manic Episode, Hypomanic Episode, Psychotic Symptoms, Panic Disorder, Generalized Anxiety Disorder [GAD], and Obsessive-Compulsive Disorder [OCD]), the interviewer is given the option of skipping to Module J to determine if a medical condition and/or substance/medication is the cause of the psychiatric symptoms characteristic of the diagnosed disorder. For medical conditions, the interviewer first determines whether at the time of symptom onset the subject/patient had a medical condition that is known to cause the type of psychiatric symptoms characteristic of the disorder. (A list of such medical conditions is provided on page J-2). If so, a diagnosis of a "probable" mental disorder due to a medical condition is made (and noted on the "Diagnostic Summary" score sheet) if the psychiatric symptoms occurred exclusively during those times when the subject/patient had the medical condition. For substances, medications, and toxins, the interviewer first asks if the subject/patient was using a substance or medication that is known to cause the type of psychiatric symptoms characteristic of the disorder at the time of the onset of the symptoms, according to the lists on page J-2. If so, a diagnosis of a "probable" substance/medication-induced mental disorder is made (and noted on the "Diagnostic Summary" score sheet) if the psychiatric symptoms have occurred exclusively during those times when the subject/patient was using (or withdrawing from) a substance or taking a medication. The word "probable" is used in all cases because additional investigation and clinical judgment may be required for a more definitive determination.

Special Instructions for Certain Sections

1. The assessment format on page A-15 differs from the other parts of the QuickSCID-5, reflecting the two separate components of Module A. The first component (which runs from pages A-1 through A-14) assesses for the presence of current and past Major Depressive Episode, Manic Episode, and Hypomanic Episode. The second component (confined to page A-15) uses a decision tree approach to determine the DSM-5 mood disorder diagnosis (if any) that corresponds to the pattern of episodes (e.g., Hypomanic Episode plus Major Depressive Episode without Manic Episodes means the diagnosis is Bipolar II Disorder). The interviewer navigates this page by evaluating the statement in each box of the tree and follows the outgoing arrow corresponding to whether the answer to the statement is "YES" or "NO" (see example below). Note that the bolded item codes in the questions direct the interviewer to the locations for the ratings made earlier in the interview.

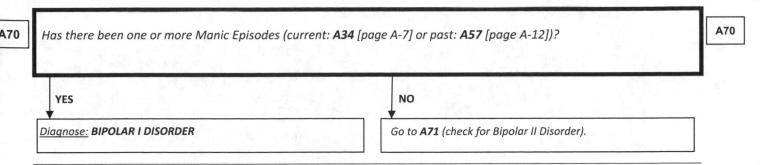

A70 | *Has there been one or more Manic Episodes (current: **A34** [page A-7] or past: **A57** [page A-12])?* | **A70**

YES

NO

<u>Diagnose:</u> **BIPOLAR I DISORDER**

Go to **A71** (check for Bipolar II Disorder).

2. Episodes of elevated or irritable mood lasting 4–6 days (thus too brief to be manic episodes) that cause severe impairment in functioning (thus too severe to be hypomanic episodes) are diagnosed in DSM-5 as Other Specified Bipolar and Related Disorder. To simplify the diagnostic flow, the QuickSCID-5 considers these severe 4- to 6-day episodes to be manic episodes.

3. Module B screens for the lifetime occurrence of delusions and hallucinations with questions likely to elicit false positive answers. Consequently, it is recommended that the interviewer ask for examples and rate "+" only if the answer is clearly indicative of psychosis. In such cases, the interviewer should also determine if the symptom has been present during the last month by asking, "Have you been experiencing this during the last month?" As noted at the top of page B-1, items should be rated "+" only if the symptoms are not caused by a medical condition or a substance. (The questions in Module J can be used to assist with this determination.)

4. Module C assesses for Alcohol and Other Substance Use Disorders during the past 12 months. The assessment for Alcohol Use Disorder can be skipped if the subject/patient has drunk alcohol fewer than six times in the past 12 months. (Note that "six times" refers to six different times over the past 12 months and not "six drinks" at any one time.) The Nonalcohol Substance Use Disorder section begins with a screen for use of different drug classes during the past 12 months. For recreational drugs, the drug class should be rated "+" if the subject/patient reports using the drug on at least several occasions during the past 12 months. For prescribed drugs, the drug class should be rated "+" if there is evidence that the prescribed drug was being abused (e.g., taking more than prescribed). If the subject/patient reports significant use of substances from more than one drug class in the past 12 months, the interviewer should start with the drug class reported to have caused the most problems or the drug class used the most. If there are not enough items rated "+" to diagnose a Substance Use Disorder for that drug class and the pattern of use of another drug class also seems problematic, the interviewer should repeat the 11 substance use questions for the additional problematic drug class.

5. The "Diagnostic Summary" score sheet at the beginning of the QuickSCID-5 is filled out at the conclusion of the interview. Item codes and page numbers on the score sheet indicate where within the body of the QuickSCID-5 the diagnoses were made.

OVERVIEW (OPTIONAL)

How old are you?
Who do you live with? (What kind of place do you live in?)

What kind of work do you do?

Are you currently working (getting paid)?

How many hours do you typically work each week?

   IF NOT WORKING: **How are you supporting yourself now?**

   IF UNKNOWN: **Has there ever been a period of time when you were unable to work or go to school?**

    IF YES: **Why was that?**

HISTORY OF CURRENT ILLNESS

What's the major problem you've been having?

Are you currently seeing a doctor, a therapist, or a counselor for help with your problem?

   IF YES: **What kind of help did you receive?**

    Counseling or psychotherapy? Medication—what kind?

What was going on in your life when this began?

When were you last feeling OK (your usual self)?

PAST PSYCHIATRIC HISTORY

When was the first time you saw someone for emotional or psychiatric problems? (What was that for? What treatment[s] did you receive? What medications?)

Have you been in treatment since then?

Have you ever been a patient in a psychiatric hospital or a psychiatric unit in a medical hospital?

Have you ever had any treatment for drugs or alcohol?

MEDICAL PROBLEMS

How has your physical health been? (Have you had any medical problems?)

Have you ever been in a hospital for treatment of a medical problem? (What was that for?)

Do you take any medications, vitamins, or other nutritional supplements (other than those you've already told me about)?

SUICIDAL IDEATION AND BEHAVIOR (This section can be skipped if a suicide rating scale is being used.)

Have you ever wished you were dead or wished you could go to sleep and not wake up?

    IF YES: **Did you have any of these thoughts in the past week (including today)?**

Have you had a strong urge to kill yourself at any time in the past week?

In the past week, did you have any thoughts of attempting suicide?

In the past week, have you thought about <u>how</u> you might actually kill yourself?

    IF YES: **Have you thought about what you would need to do to carry this out? Do you have the means to do this?**

Have you ever tried to kill yourself?

    IF NO: **Have you ever done anything to harm yourself? Were you trying to end your life?**

A. MOOD EPISODES AND DISORDERS

	CURRENT MAJOR DEPRESSIVE EPISODE			
A1	For the past 2 weeks, have you been feeling depressed, down, sad, empty, or hopeless, for most of the day, nearly every day?	–	+	**A1**
A2	For the past 2 weeks, have you lost interest or pleasure in things you usually enjoyed, for most of the day, nearly every day?	–	+	**A2**
	*If **A1** and **A2** are BOTH coded "–," skip to **A12** (Past Major Depressive Episode), **page A-3**. Otherwise, continue with **A3**, below.*			
A3	For the past 2 weeks, has your appetite been decreased or increased, nearly every day? **Did you lose or gain weight without trying to, by at least** (5% OF PERSON'S BODY WEIGHT) **in a month?**	–	+	**A3**
A4	In the past 2 weeks, did you have trouble falling asleep or staying asleep, waking frequently or waking too early, nearly every night? **How about sleeping too much, nearly every night?**	–	+	**A4**
A5	In the past 2 weeks, have you been so fidgety or restless that you couldn't sit still, so that other people noticed it, nearly every day? **What about the opposite—talking more slowly or moving more slowly than is normal for you, as if you're moving through molasses or mud, so that other people noticed it, nearly every day?**	–	+	**A5**
A6	In the past 2 weeks, were you tired all the time or was your energy very low, nearly every day?	–	+	**A6**
A7	In the past 2 weeks, have you been feeling worthless nearly every day? **What about feeling guilty about things you have done or not done, nearly every day (not including feeling guilty about not taking care of things because you have been sick)?**	–	+	**A7**
A8	In the past 2 weeks, have you had trouble thinking or concentrating nearly every day? **Has it been hard to make decisions about everyday things nearly every day?**	–	+	**A8**

A9 In the past 2 weeks, have things been so bad that you thought a lot about death or that you would be better off dead?   −   +   A9

Have you thought about taking your own life?

Have you made a specific plan? Have you done anything to prepare for it?

Have you actually tried to kill yourself?

If fewer than five items (A1–A9) are coded "+," skip to A12 (Past Major Depressive Episode), page A-3. Otherwise, continue with A10.

A10 Have these problems made it difficult for you to do your work, take care of things at home, or get along with other people?   −   +   A1

Are you very bothered by the fact that you have these symptoms?

Skip to A12 (Past Major Depressive Episode), page A-3.

CURRENT MAJOR DEPRESSIVE EPISODE

IF A CONCURRENT MEDICAL CONDITION OR SUBSTANCE/MEDICATION USE, SKIP TO MODULE J TO RULE OUT DEPRESSIVE DISORDER DUE TO ANOTHER MEDICAL CONDITION AND/OR SUBSTANCE-INDUCED DEPRESSIVE DISORDER AND THEN RETURN HERE.

Continue with A11, below.

A11 How many separate times in your life have you been depressed or lost interest in things nearly every day for at least 2 weeks and had several of the symptoms of depression that you just told me about?   ___ ___   A11

Skip to A23 (Current Manic Episode), page A-5.

	PAST MAJOR DEPRESSIVE EPISODE		
	*Note: If there currently is depressed mood or loss of interest but full criteria are not met for a current Major Depressive Episode, substitute the phrase "Has there ever been __another__ time ..." for both of the below questions (i.e., **A12** and **A13**).*		
A12	Have you <u>ever</u> had a time when you were feeling depressed, down, sad, empty, or hopeless, for most of the day, nearly every day, <u>for at least 2 weeks</u>?	– +	**A12**
A13	➤ *IF PREVIOUS ITEM RATED "+":* During that time, did you also lose interest or pleasure in things you usually enjoyed nearly every day? ➤ *IF PREVIOUS ITEM RATED "–":* Have you <u>ever</u> had a period of time when you lost interest or pleasure in things you usually enjoyed, nearly every day, that lasted <u>for at least 2 weeks</u>?	– +	**A13**
	*If **A12** and **A13** are <u>BOTH</u> coded "–," skip to **A23** (Current Manic Episode), **page A-5**. Otherwise, continue below.*		
	Have you had more than one time like that? IF YES: Which time was the worst?	*Indicate month/year of onset of worst episode:* _____	
	During that time when you (were depressed AND/OR **lost interest in things**), when were you feeling the worst?		
A14	Focusing on the worst 2 weeks during that time ... ... was your appetite decreased or increased, nearly every day? ... did you lose or gain weight without trying to, by at least (5% OF PERSON'S BODY WEIGHT) in a month?	– +	**A14**
A15	... did you have trouble falling asleep or staying asleep, or waking frequently, or waking too early, nearly every night? ... were you sleeping too much, nearly every night?	– +	**A15**

A16	Focusing on the worst 2 weeks during that time … … were you so fidgety or restless that you couldn't sit still, so that other people noticed it, nearly every day? What about the opposite—were you talking more slowly or moving more slowly than was normal for you, as if you were moving through molasses or mud, so that other people noticed it, nearly every day?	– +
A17	… were you tired all the time or was your energy very low, nearly every day?	– +
A18	… did you feel worthless nearly every day? … did you feel guilty about things you had done or not done, nearly every day (not including feeling guilty about not taking care of things because you have been sick)?	– +
A19	… did you have trouble thinking or concentrating nearly every day? … was it hard to make decisions about everyday things nearly every day?	– +
A20	… were things so bad that you thought a lot about death or that you would be better off dead? Did you think about taking your own life? Did you make a specific plan? Did you do anything to prepare for it? Did you actually try to kill yourself?	– +

If fewer than five items (A12–A20) are coded "+," skip to A23 (Current Manic Episode), page A-5. Otherwise, continue with A21, below.

A21	Did these problems make it difficult for you to do your work, take care of things at home, or get along with other people? Were you very bothered by the fact that you had these symptoms?	– ↓ + ↓ *Skip to A23 (Current Manic Episode), page A-5.* **PAST MAJOR DEPRESSIVE EPISODE**
	*IF A CONCURRENT MEDICAL CONDITION OR SUBSTANCE/MEDICATION USE, SKIP TO **MODULE J** TO RULE OUT DEPRESSIVE DISORDER DUE TO ANOTHER MEDICAL CONDITION AND/OR SUBSTANCE-INDUCED DEPRESSIVE DISORDER AND THEN RETURN HERE.*	
		Continue with A22, below.
A22	How many separate times in your life have you been depressed or lost interest in things nearly every day for at least 2 weeks and had several of the symptoms of depression that you just told me about?	___ ___

CURRENT MANIC EPISODE

A23 | Over the past few days, have you been feeling so good, "high," excited, or "on top of the world" that other people thought you were not your normal self? Was that more than just feeling good?

    IF YES: Have you also felt like you were "hyper" or "wired" and had an unusual amount of energy or that you were much more active than is typical for you?

Note: Code "+" only if "YES" to both elevated mood and increased energy.

−   +   **A23**

Skip to A25.

Continue with A24.

A24 | Over the past few days, have you been feeling irritable, angry, or short-tempered for most of the day, for at least several days, in a way that is different from the way you usually are?

    IF YES: Have you also felt like you were "hyper" or "wired" and had an unusual amount of energy or that you were much more active than is typical for you?

Note: Code "+" only if "YES" to both irritable mood and increased energy.

−   +   **A24**

Continue with A25.

Skip to A46 (Past Manic Episode), page A-10.

A25 | Have you been feeling (**high** AND/OR **irritable**) and full of energy nearly every day for at least 1 week? | −   + | **A25**

A26 | Have you needed to go into the hospital to be protected from hurting yourself or someone else or from doing something that could have caused serious financial or legal problems? | −   + | **A26**

*If **A25** and **A26** are BOTH coded "−," skip to **A35** (Current Hypomanic Episode), **page A-8**. Otherwise, continue below.*

A27 | During this time when you have been (**high** AND/OR **irritable**) …

… have you been much more self-confident than usual?

Compared with how you usually feel, have you felt much smarter or better than everyone else or that you have special powers or abilities? | −   + | **A27**

A28 | … have you needed much less sleep than usual, and yet you still have felt rested? | −   + | **A28**

A29	**While you have been** (**high** AND/OR **irritable**), … **have you been much more talkative than usual?** … **have people had trouble stopping you or understanding you or had trouble getting a word in edgewise?**	− +	A29
A30	… **have your thoughts been racing through your head?**	− +	A30
A31	… **have you been so easily distracted by things going on around you that you have had trouble concentrating or staying on one track?**	− +	A31
A32	… **have you been much more productive or spending much more time at work or school, as compared to usual?** … **have you been much more sociable, such as calling or going out with friends more than you usually would, or have you been making a lot of new friends?** … **have you been spending much more time thinking about sex or being sexually active, either by yourself or with others, as compared with how you usually are?** … **have you been physically restless during this time, doing things like pacing a lot or being unable to sit still?** *Note: Code "+" if "YES" to any of these questions.*	− +	A32
A33	… **have you done potentially risky things without considering how they might hurt you or get you into trouble?** **Things like …** … **going on wild buying sprees or gambling with money you couldn't afford to lose?** … **making foolish business investments or getting involved in unwise business schemes?** … **engaging in sexual behavior that wouldn't be usual for you that could have gotten (or did get) you into trouble?**	− +	A33

*If manic mood was euphoric (**A23** coded "+"):* If fewer than *three* items (**A27–A33**) are coded "+," skip to **A46** *(Past Manic Episode)* **page A-10.** Otherwise, continue with **A34**.

*If manic mood was irritable but not euphoric (**A24** coded "+" but **A23** coded "–"):* If fewer than *four* items (**A27–A33**) are coded "+," skip to **A46** *(Past Manic Episode)* **page A-10.** Otherwise, continue with **A34**.

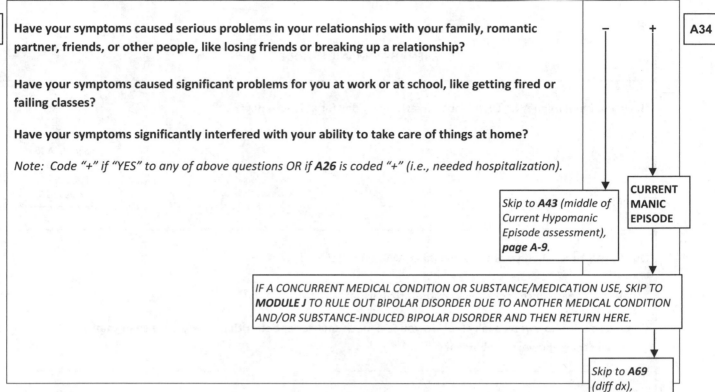

A34

Have your symptoms caused serious problems in your relationships with your family, romantic partner, friends, or other people, like losing friends or breaking up a relationship?

Have your symptoms caused significant problems for you at work or at school, like getting fired or failing classes?

Have your symptoms significantly interfered with your ability to take care of things at home?

*Note: Code "+" if "YES" to any of above questions OR if **A26** is coded "+" (i.e., needed hospitalization).*

      −   +   **A34**

*Skip to **A43** (middle of Current Hypomanic Episode assessment), **page A-9**.*

CURRENT MANIC EPISODE

*IF A CONCURRENT MEDICAL CONDITION OR SUBSTANCE/MEDICATION USE, SKIP TO **MODULE J** TO RULE OUT BIPOLAR DISORDER DUE TO ANOTHER MEDICAL CONDITION AND/OR SUBSTANCE-INDUCED BIPOLAR DISORDER AND THEN RETURN HERE.*

*Skip to **A69** (diff dx), **page A-15**.*

	CURRENT HYPOMANIC EPISODE		
A35	Have you been (**high** AND/OR **irritable**) nearly every day for at least 4 days?	– *Skip to **A46** (Past Manic Episode) page A-10.*	+	A35
A36	During this time when you have been (**high** AND/OR **irritable**) … … have you been much more self-confident than usual? Compared with how you usually feel, do you feel much smarter or better than everyone else or that you have special powers or abilities?	–	+	A36
A37	… have you needed much less sleep than usual, and yet you still feel rested?	–	+	A37
A38	… have you been much more talkative than usual? … have people had trouble stopping you or understanding you or had trouble getting a word in edgewise?	–	+	A38
A39	… have your thoughts been racing through your head?	–	+	A39
A40	… have you been so easily distracted by things going on around you that you have had trouble concentrating or staying on one track?	–	+	A40
A41	… have you been much more productive or spending more time at work or school, as compared to usual? … have you been much more sociable, such as calling or going out with friends more than you usually would, or have you been making a lot of new friends? … have you been spending much more time thinking about sex or being sexually active, either by yourself or with others, as compared to usual? … have you been physically restless during this time, doing things like pacing a lot or being unable to sit still? *Note: Code "+" if "YES" to any of these questions.*	–	+	A41

A42	**During this time when you have been (high** AND/OR **irritable) …** **… have you been doing potentially risky things without considering how they might hurt you or get you into trouble?** **Things like …** **… going on wild buying sprees or gambling with money you couldn't afford to lose?** **… making foolish business investments or getting involved in unwise business schemes?** **… engaging in sexual behavior that wouldn't be usual for you that could have gotten (or did get) you into trouble?**	– + **A42**

*If hypomanic mood was euphoric (**A23** coded "+"): If fewer than <u>three</u> items (**A36–A42**) are coded "+," skip to **A46** (Past Manic Episode), **page A-10**. Otherwise, continue with **A43**.*

*If hypomanic mood was irritable but not euphoric (**A24** coded "+" but **A23** coded "–"): If fewer than <u>four</u> items (**A36–A42**) are coded "+," skip to **A46** (Past Manic Episode), **page A-10**. Otherwise, continue with **A43**.*

A43	**Has this period of being (high** AND/OR **irritable) been very different from the way you usually are?**	– + **A43**
A44	**Have other people noticed this change in you?**	– + **A44**

*If **A43** and **A44** are BOTH coded "–." skip to **A46** (Past Manic Episode), **page A-10**. Otherwise continue with **A45**.*

A45	**Have your symptoms caused serious problems in your relationships with your family, romantic partner, friends, or other people, like losing friends or breaking up a relationship?** **Have your symptoms caused significant problems for you at work or at school, like getting fired or failing classes?** **Have your symptoms significantly interfered with your ability to take care of things at home?** *Note: If "YES" to any of these questions, impairment is too severe to be considered a Hypomanic Episode. Code "+" and go back to **A34** and diagnose Current Manic Episode.*	– + **A45**

*Go back to **A34** (impairment assessment for Current Manic Episode) and code **A34** "+," page A-7.*

CURRENT HYPOMANIC EPISODE

*IF A CONCURRENT MEDICAL CONDITION OR SUBSTANCE/MEDICATION USE, SKIP TO **MODULE J** TO RULE OUT BIPOLAR DISORDER DUE TO ANOTHER MEDICAL CONDITION AND/OR SUBSTANCE-INDUCED BIPOLAR DISORDER AND THEN RETURN HERE.*

*Continue with **A46** (Past Manic Episode), **page A-10**.*

PAST MANIC EPISODE

A46	Have you <u>ever</u> had a time when you were feeling so good, "high," excited, or "on top of the world" that other people thought you were not your normal self? Was that more than just feeling good? IF YES: **Did you also feel like you were "hyper" or "wired" and had an unusual amount of energy or that you were much more active than is typical for you?** *Note: Code "+" only if "YES" to both elevated mood and increased energy.*	– + *Skip to* ***A48.*** *Continue with* ***A47.***	**A46**
A47	Have you <u>ever</u> had a period of time when you were feeling irritable, angry, or short-tempered for most of the day, for at least several days, and that was different from the way you usually are? IF YES: **Did you also feel like you were "hyper" or "wired" and had an unusual amount of energy or that you were much more active than is typical for you?** *Note: Code "+" only if "YES" to both irritable mood and increased energy.*	– + *Continue with* ***A48.*** *Skip to* ***A69*** *(diff dx),* ***page A-15.***	**A47**
A48	Were you (**high** AND/OR **irritable**) and full of energy nearly every day for at least 1 week?	– +	**A48**
A49	During this period of time, did you need to go into the hospital to be protected from hurting yourself or someone else or from doing something that could have caused serious financial or legal problems?	– +	**A49**

*If **A48** and **A49** are BOTH coded "–," skip to **A68** (Past Hypomanic Episode), **page A-14.** Otherwise, continue below.*

	Have you had more than one time like that? *IF YES:* **Which time was the most intense or caused the most problems?**	Indicate month/year of onset of worst episode: _____	
A50	**During that time …** **… were you much more self-confident than usual?** **Compared with how you usually felt, did you feel much smarter or better than everyone else or that you had special powers or abilities?**	– +	**A50**

		−	+	
A51	During that time … … did you need much less sleep than usual, and yet you still felt rested?	−	+	A51
A52	… were you much more talkative than usual? … did people have trouble stopping you or understanding you or have trouble getting a word in edgewise?	−	+	A52
A53	… were your thoughts racing through your head?	−	+	A53
A54	… were you so easily distracted by things going on around you that you had trouble concentrating or staying on one track?	−	+	A54
A55	… were you much more productive or spending much more time at work or school as compared to usual? … were you much more sociable during that time, such as calling or going out with friends more than you usually would, or were you making a lot of new friends? … were you spending much more time thinking about sex or being sexually active, either by yourself or with others, as compared to usual? … were you physically restless during this time, doing things like pacing a lot or being unable to sit still? *Note: Code "+" if "YES" to any of these questions.*	−	+	A55
A56	… did you do potentially risky things without considering how they might hurt you or get you into trouble? Things like … … going on wild buying sprees or gambling with money you couldn't afford to lose? … making foolish business investments or getting involved in unwise business schemes? … engaging in sexual behavior that wouldn't be usual for you that could have gotten (or did get) you into trouble? … did you engage in activities without considering potential risks or negative consequences for you or your family?	−	+	A56

*If manic mood was euphoric (**A46** coded "+"): If fewer than three items (**A50–A56**) are coded "+," skip to **next module**. Otherwise, continue with **A57**.*

*If manic mood was irritable but not euphoric (**A47** coded "+" but **A46** coded "−"): If fewer than four items (**A50–A56**) are coded "+," skip to **next module**. Otherwise, continue with **A57**.*

A57 | **Did your symptoms cause serious problems in your relationships with your family, romantic partner, friends, or other people, like losing friends or breaking up a relationship?**

Did your symptoms cause significant problems for you at work or at school, like getting fired or failing classes?

Did your symptoms significantly interfere with your ability to take care of things at home?

Note: Code "+" if "YES" to any of these questions OR if A49 is coded "+" (i.e., needed hospitalization).

–   +   **A57**

Skip to A66 (middle of Past Hypo-manic Episode assessment), page A-14.

PAST MANIC EPISODE

IF A CONCURRENT MEDICAL CONDITION OR SUBSTANCE/MEDICATION USE, SKIP TO **MODULE J** TO RULE OUT BIPOLAR DISORDER DUE TO ANOTHER MEDICAL CONDITION AND/OR SUBSTANCE-INDUCED BIPOLAR DISORDER AND THEN RETURN HERE.

Skip to A69 (diff dx), page A-15.

PAST HYPOMANIC EPISODE

A58	Were you (**high** AND/OR **irritable**) nearly every day for at least 4 days?	− + **A58**
		↓ *Skip to **A69** (diff dx), **page A-15**.*
	Have you had more than one time like that? *IF YES:* **Which time was the most intense or caused the most problems?**	*Indicate month/year of onset of worst episode:* _____
A59	**During that time …** **… were you much more self-confident than usual?** **Compared with how you usually feel, did you feel much smarter or better than everyone else or that you had special powers or abilities?**	− + **A59**
A60	**… did you need much less sleep than usual, and yet you still felt rested?**	− + **A60**
A61	**… were you much more talkative than usual?** **… did people have trouble stopping you or understanding you or have trouble getting a word in edgewise?**	− + **A61**
A62	**… were your thoughts racing through your head?**	− + **A62**
A63	**… were you so easily distracted by things going on around you that you had trouble concentrating or staying on one track?**	− + **A63**
A64	**… were you much more productive or spending much more time at work as compared to usual?** **… were you much more sociable during that time, such as calling or going out with friends more than you usually would, or were you making a lot of new friends?** **… were you spending much more time thinking about sex or being more sexually active, either by yourself or with others, as compared to usual?** **… were you physically restless during this time, doing things like pacing a lot or being unable to sit still?** *Note: Code "+" if "YES" to any of these questions.*	− + **A64**

| A65 | During that time, did you do potentially risky things without considering how they might hurt you or get you into trouble?

Things like …

… going on wild buying sprees, or gambling with money you couldn't afford to lose?

… making foolish business investments or getting involved in unwise business schemes?

… engaging in sexual behavior that wouldn't be usual for you that could have gotten (or did get) you into trouble?? | –   + | A65 |

*If hypomanic mood was euphoric (A46 coded "+"): If fewer than <u>three</u> items (A59–A65) are coded "+," skip to **next module**. Otherwise, continue with A66.*

*If hypomanic mood was irritable but not euphoric (A47 coded "+" but A46 coded "–"): If fewer than <u>four</u> items (A59–A65) are coded "+," skip to **next module**. Otherwise, continue with A66.*

| A66 | Was this period of being (high AND/OR irritable) very different from the way you usually are? | –   + | A66 |
| A67 | Did other people notice this change in you? | –   + | A67 |

If A66 and A67 are BOTH coded "–." skip to A69 (diff dx), page A-15. Otherwise continue with A68.

| A68 | Did your symptoms cause serious problems in your relationships with your family, romantic partner, friends, or other people, like losing friends or breaking up a relationship?

Did your symptoms cause significant problems for you at work or at school, like getting fired or failing classes?

Did your symptoms significantly interfere with your ability to take care of things at home?

Note: Code "+" if "YES" to any of these questions OR if **A49** (i.e., needed hospitalization) is coded "+."

Note: If "YES" to any of these questions, impairment is too severe to be considered a Hypomanic Episode. Code "+" and go back to **A57** and diagnose Past Manic Episode. | –   + | A68 |

Go back to A57 (impairment assessment for Past Manic Episode) and code A57 "+," page A-12.

PAST HYPOMANIC EPISODE

*IF A CONCURRENT MEDICAL CONDITION OR SUBSTANCE/MEDICATION USE, SKIP TO **MODULE J** TO RULE OUT BIPOLAR DISORDER DUE TO ANOTHER MEDICAL CONDITION AND/OR SUBSTANCE-INDUCED BIPOLAR DISORDER AND THEN RETURN HERE.*

Continue with A69 (diff dx), page A-15.

DIFFERENTIAL DIAGNOSIS OF MOOD DISORDERS

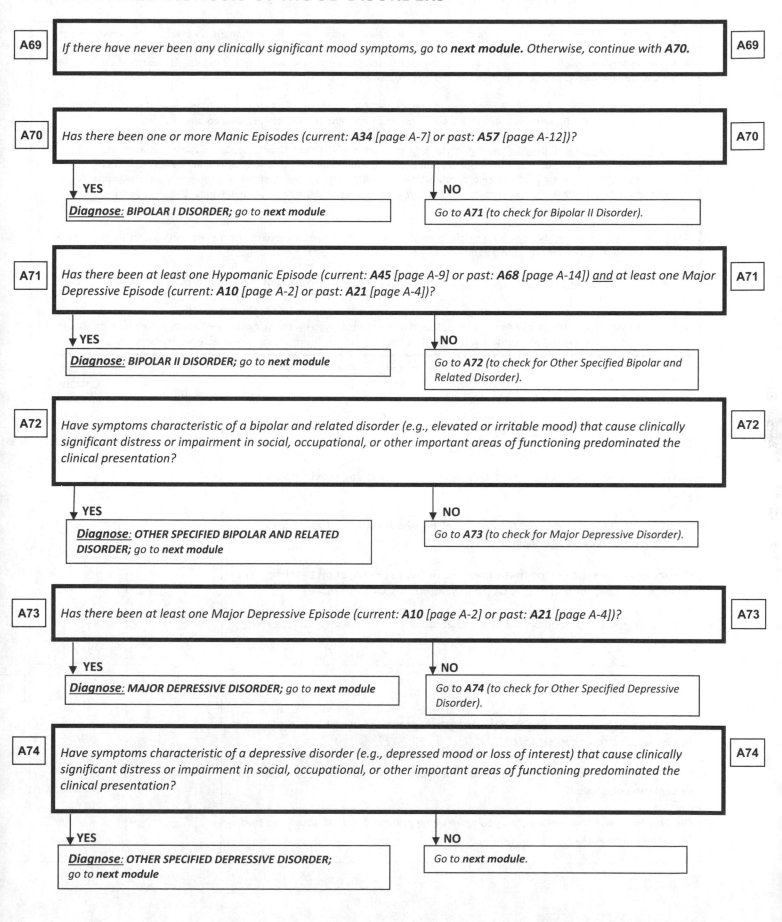

A69 | If there have never been any clinically significant mood symptoms, go to **next module**. Otherwise, continue with **A70**. | **A69**

A70 | Has there been one or more Manic Episodes (current: **A34** [page A-7] or past: **A57** [page A-12])? | **A70**

YES

Diagnose: BIPOLAR I DISORDER; go to **next module**

NO

Go to **A71** (to check for Bipolar II Disorder).

A71 | Has there been at least one Hypomanic Episode (current: **A45** [page A-9] or past: **A68** [page A-14]) <u>and</u> at least one Major Depressive Episode (current: **A10** [page A-2] or past: **A21** [page A-4])? | **A71**

YES

Diagnose: BIPOLAR II DISORDER; go to **next module**

NO

Go to **A72** (to check for Other Specified Bipolar and Related Disorder).

A72 | Have symptoms characteristic of a bipolar and related disorder (e.g., elevated or irritable mood) that cause clinically significant distress or impairment in social, occupational, or other important areas of functioning predominated the clinical presentation? | **A72**

YES

Diagnose: OTHER SPECIFIED BIPOLAR AND RELATED DISORDER; go to **next module**

NO

Go to **A73** (to check for Major Depressive Disorder).

A73 | Has there been at least one Major Depressive Episode (current: **A10** [page A-2] or past: **A21** [page A-4])? | **A73**

YES

Diagnose: MAJOR DEPRESSIVE DISORDER; go to **next module**

NO

Go to **A74** (to check for Other Specified Depressive Disorder).

A74 | Have symptoms characteristic of a depressive disorder (e.g., depressed mood or loss of interest) that cause clinically significant distress or impairment in social, occupational, or other important areas of functioning predominated the clinical presentation? | **A74**

YES

Diagnose: OTHER SPECIFIED DEPRESSIVE DISORDER; go to **next module**

NO

Go to **next module**.

B. PSYCHOTIC SYMPTOM SCREEN

> *For any psychotic symptom concurrent with a substance/medication/toxin or medical condition listed below, determine whether the symptom is primary or else better explained by a substance ([I] = during intoxication, [W] = during withdrawal, [I/W] = during intoxication or withdrawal), a medication, a toxin, or a medical condition using the questions in Module J for guidance. Code "+" only if primary (i.e., not due to medical condition or substance induced).*
>
> <u>Substances known to cause psychotic symptoms include</u> alcohol (I/W); cannabis (I); hallucinogens (I), phencyclidine and related substances (I); inhalants (I); sedatives, hypnotics, and anxiolytics (I/W); and stimulants (including cocaine) (I).
>
> <u>Medications known to cause psychotic symptoms include</u> anesthetics and analgesics; anticholinergic agents; anticonvulsants; antihistamines; antihypertensive and cardiovascular medications; antimicrobial medications; antiparkinsonian medications; chemotherapeutic agents (e.g., cyclosporine, procarbazine); corticosteroids; gastrointestinal medications; muscle relaxants; nonsteroidal anti-inflammatory medications; other over-the-counter medications (e.g., phenylephrine, pseudoephedrine); antidepressant medication; and disulfiram.
>
> <u>Toxins known to cause psychotic symptoms include</u> anticholinesterases, organophosphate insecticides, sarin and other nerve gases, carbon monoxide, carbon dioxide, and volatile substances such as fuel or paint.
>
> <u>Medical conditions known to cause psychotic symptoms include</u> neurological conditions (e.g., neoplasms, cerebrovascular disease, Huntington's disease, multiple sclerosis, epilepsy, auditory or visual nerve injury or impairment, deafness, migraine, central nervous system infections), endocrine conditions (e.g., hyper- and hypothyroidism, hyper- and hypoparathyroidism, hyper- and hypoadrenocorticism), metabolic conditions (e.g., hypoxia, hypercarbia, hypoglycemia), fluid or electrolyte imbalances, hepatic or renal diseases, and autoimmune disorders with central nervous system involvement (e.g., systemic lupus erythematosus).

		Lifetime		Current (Past Month)		
B1	*Delusions of reference* **Has it ever seemed like people were talking about you or taking special notice of you?** *IF YES:* **Were you convinced they were talking about you or did you think it might have been your imagination?** **Did you ever have the feeling that something on TV, the radio, or on a website was meant specifically for you or was trying to send you a special message?** **Did you ever have the feeling that street signs or billboards had a special meaning for you?**	–	+	–	+	**B1**
B2	*Persecutory delusions* **Have you ever had the feeling that you were being followed, watched, spied on, or put under electronic surveillance?** **Have you ever had the feeling that people were plotting or conspiring to harm you or someone you loved?** **Did you ever have the feeling that you were being poisoned or that your food had been tampered with?**	–	+	–	+	**B2**

		Lifetime		Current (Past Month)		
B3	*Grandiose delusions* **Have you ever felt that you were especially important, powerful, wealthy, or famous?** **Have you ever felt like you had special powers such as being able to read minds or predict the future?** **Did you ever believe that you had a special or close relationship with God, a deity, or someone famous?**	–	+	–	+	**B3**
B4	*Somatic delusions* **Have you ever felt that your organs or other parts of your body were somehow diseased, abnormal, or changed?** **Have you ever been convinced that something was very wrong with your physical health even though your doctor said nothing was wrong ... like you had cancer or some other disease?**	–	+	–	+	**B4**
B5	*Delusions of guilt* **Have you ever felt that you had committed a crime or done something terrible for which you should be punished?** **Have you ever felt that something you did, or should have done but did not do, caused serious harm to your parents, children, other family members, or friends?**	–	+	–	+	**B5**
B6	*Religious delusions* **Have you ever felt that God, the devil, or some other spiritual being or higher power has communicated directly with you?** *IF YES:* **Do others in your religious or spiritual community also have such experiences?** *Code "+" only if yes to the first question and "NO" to the second question about others also having such experiences.*	–	+	–	+	**B6**

		Lifetime	Current (Past Month)	
B7	*Delusions of being controlled* **Did you ever feel that someone or something outside yourself was controlling your thoughts or actions against your will?**	– +	– +	**B7**
B8	*Thought insertion/withdrawal* **Did you ever feel that certain thoughts that were not your own were put into your head or that your own thoughts were being taken out of your head?**	– +	– +	**B8**
B9	*Thought broadcasting* **Did you ever feel as if your thoughts were being broadcast out loud so that other people could read your thoughts?**	– +	– +	**B9**
B10	*Other delusions* **Have you ever had any thoughts that you believed to be true that others told you were not true?**	– +	– +	**B10**
B11	*Auditory hallucinations* **Did you ever hear things that other people couldn't, such as noises or the voices of people whispering or talking?**	– +	– +	**B11**
B12	*Visual hallucinations* **Did you ever have visions or see things that other people couldn't see?** *IF YES:* **Has this happened only when you are falling asleep or waking up?** *Note: Code "–" if only happens during falling asleep or awakening.*	– +	– +	**B12**
B13	*If any psychotic symptom in lifetime column is rated "+," then check here ___ (**POSSIBLE LIFETIME PSYCHOTIC DISORDER**).*			**B13**
B14	*If any psychotic symptom in current column is rated "+," then check here ___ (**POSSIBLE CURRENT PSYCHOTIC DISORDER**).*			**B14**

Continue with **next module**.

C. ALCOHOL AND OTHER SUBSTANCE USE DISORDERS

	PAST-12-MONTH ALCOHOL USE DISORDER		
C1	Have you drunk alcohol at least six times in the past 12 months, since (12 MONTHS AGO)?	–	+	**C1**
	Skip to C14 (Nonalcohol Substance Use Disorder), page C-4.		
	I'd like to ask you some more questions about your drinking habits in the past 12 months.		
C2	During the past 12 months … … have you found that once you started drinking you ended up drinking much more than you intended to? For example, you planned to have only one or two drinks, but you ended up having many more? What about drinking for a much longer period of time than you intended?	–	+	**C2**
C3	… have you repeatedly wanted to stop, cut down, or control your drinking? … have you tried to stop, cut down, or control your drinking but failed?	–	+	**C3**
C4	… on those days when you were drinking, did you spend a great deal of time drinking, being drunk, or hung over?	–	+	**C4**
C5	… have you had a strong desire or urge to drink in between those times when you were drinking?	–	+	**C5**
C6	… have you missed work or school or often arrived late because you were intoxicated, high, or very hung over? How about … … doing a bad job at work or school, or failing courses, or getting kicked out of school because of your drinking? … getting into trouble at work or school because of your use of alcohol? … not taking care of things at home because of your drinking, like paying bills, making sure food and clean clothes are available for your family, and making sure your children go to school and get medical care?	–	+	**C6**

C7	**During the past 12 months, since** (12 MONTHS AGO), … **… has your drinking caused problems with other people, such as family members, friends, or people at work?** *IF YES*: **Did you keep on drinking anyway?** *Note: Code "+" only if "YES" to both questions.*	–	+	**C7**
C8	**… have you had to give up or reduce the time you spent at work or school, with family or friends, or doing things you like to do because you were drinking or hung over?**	–	+	**C8**
C9	**… have you repeatedly had a few drinks right before doing something that requires coordination and concentration like driving, boating, climbing on a ladder, or operating heavy machinery?** *IF YES*: **Would you say that the amount you had to drink affected your coordination or concentration so that it was more likely that you or someone else could have been hurt?** *Note: Code "+" only if "YES" to both questions.*	–	+	**C9**
C10	**… has your drinking caused you any problems like making you very depressed or anxious, making it difficult for you to sleep, or making it so you couldn't later recall what happened while you were drinking?** **… has your drinking caused significant physical problems or made a physical problem, such as stomach ulcers, liver disease, or pancreatitis, worse?** *IF YES TO EITHER OF ABOVE*: **Did you keep on drinking anyway?** *Note: Code "+" only if "YES" to both parts.*	–	+	**C10**
C11	**… have you found that you needed to drink much more than you did when you first started drinking to get the feeling you wanted or that when you drank the same amount, it had much less effect than before?**	–	+	**C11**

C12

... when you cut down or stopped drinking after a period of heavy drinking or drinking over several days, did you have at least two withdrawal symptoms, such as

    ... sweating or a racing heart?
    ... your hand[s] shaking?
    ... trouble sleeping?
    ... feeling nauseated or vomiting?
    ... seeing, feeling, or hearing things that weren't really there?
    ... feeling agitated?
    ... feeling anxious?
    ... having a seizure?

IF NONE OR ONLY ONE OF THE ABOVE SYMPTOMS: **During the past year, have you ever started the day with a drink, or did you often drink or take some other drug or medication to keep yourself from getting the shakes or becoming sick?**

−   +

C12

C13

*If at least <u>two</u> items (**C2–C12**) are coded "+":*

<u>*Diagnose*</u>:
___ ***Mild Alcohol Use Disorder*** *(if 2–3 symptoms), or*
___ ***Moderate Alcohol Use Disorder*** *(if 4–5 symptoms), or*
___ ***Severe Alcohol Use Disorder*** *(if 6 or more symptoms).*

*and continue with **C14** (Nonalcohol Substance Use Disorder).*

*Otherwise, continue with **C14** (Nonalcohol Substance Use Disorder).*

C13

PAST-12-MONTH NONALCOHOL SUBSTANCE USE DISORDER

C14	Now I'd like to ask you about your use of drugs and medicines over the past 12 months, since (12 MONTHS AGO).	**C14**	
C15	*Sedatives, Hypnotics, or Anxiolytics*: **In the past 12 months, have you taken any pills to calm you down, help you relax, or help you sleep on at least several occasions (drugs like Valium, Xanax, Ativan, Klonopin, Ambien, Sonata, or Lunesta)?** *IF PRESCRIBED*: **How about taking more than was prescribed or running out early or having to go to more than one doctor to make sure you didn't run out?** *IF YES, specific drug(s) used:* _____	– +	C15
C16	*Cannabis:* **In the past 12 months, have you used marijuana ("cannabis," "pot," "grass," "weed"), hashish ("hash"), THC concentrates ("shatter," "wax"), K2, or "spice" on at least several occasions?** *IF YES, specific drug(s) used:* _____	– +	C16
C17	*Stimulants*: **In the past 12 months, have you used any stimulants or "uppers" to give you more energy, keep you alert, lose weight, or help you focus, on at least several occasions (drugs like speed, methamphetamine, crystal meth, "crank," Ritalin or methylphenidate, Dexedrine, Adderall or amphetamine, or prescription diet pills)? How about cocaine or "crack"?** *IF PRESCRIBED*: **How about taking more than was prescribed or running out early or having to go to more than one doctor to make sure you didn't run out?** *IF YES, specific drug(s) used:* _____	– +	C17
C18	*Opioids*: **In the past 12 months, have you ever used heroin or methadone on at least several occasions? How about prescription pain killers (drugs like morphine, codeine, Percocet, Percodan, Oxycontin, Tylox or oxycodone, Vicodin, Lortab, Lorcet or hydrocodone, or Suboxone or buprenorphine)?** *IF PRESCRIBED*: **How about taking more than was prescribed or running out early or having to go to more than one doctor to make sure you didn't run out?** *IF YES, specific drug(s) used:* _____	– +	C18
C19	*Phencyclidine (PCP) and Related Substances*: **In the past 12 months, have you ever used PCP ("angel dust," "peace pill") or ketamine ("Special K," "Vitamin K") on at least several occasions?** *IF YES, specific drug(s) used:* _____	– +	C19
C20	*Other Hallucinogens*: **In the past 12 months, have you used any drugs to "trip" or heighten your senses on at least several occasions (drugs like LSD, "acid," peyote, mescaline, "mushrooms," psilocybin, Ecstasy [MDMA, "molly"], bath salts, DMT, or other hallucinogens)?** *IF YES, specific drug(s) used:* _____	– +	C20
C21	*Inhalants*: **In the past 12 months, have you ever used glue, paint, correction fluid, gasoline, or other inhalants to get high on at least several occasions?** *IF YES, specific drug(s) used:* _____	– +	C21
C22	*Other:* **What about other drugs used on at least several occasions, like anabolic steroids, nitrous oxide (laughing gas, "whippets"), nitrites (amyl nitrite, butyl nitrite, "poppers," "snappers"), diet pills (phentermine), or over-the-counter medicine for allergies, colds, cough, or sleep?** *IF YES, specific drug(s) used:* _____	– +	C22

C23

If none of the drug classes inquired about above **(C15–C22)** *were rated "+" (i.e., none of the drugs were used on at least several occasions in the past year, or, if prescribed, respondent denies taking more than was prescribed, running out of medication early, or going to more than one doctor), skip to* **next module.**

Otherwise, ask the following questions concerning the drug classes rated "+":

Which drugs or medications caused you the most problems over the past 12 months?

Which one did you use the most or was your "drug of choice"?

Specify drug: _____

C23

I'd now like to ask you some more questions about your use of (DRUG/MEDICATION SPECIFIED ABOVE) **in the past 12 months.**

C24

During the past 12 months, since (12 MONTHS AGO), **…**

… have you found that once you started using (DRUG/MEDICATION) **you ended up using much more than you** <u>intended</u> **to? For example, you planned to have only a small amount of** (DRUG/MEDICATION), **but you ended up having much more. (Tell me about that. How often did that happen?)**

… what about using (DRUG/MEDICATION) **for a much longer period of time than you** <u>intended</u> **to?**

    –   +   **C24**

C25

… have you repeatedly wanted to stop, cut down using (DRUG/MEDICATION), **or control your use of** (DRUG/MEDICATION)?

… have you tried to cut down, stop, or control your use of (DRUG/MEDICATION) **but failed?**

    –   +   **C25**

C26

… have you spent a lot of time getting (DRUG/MEDICATION) **or using** (DRUG/MEDICATION), **or has it taken a lot of time for you to get over the effects of** (DRUG/MEDICATION)?

    –   +   **C26**

C27

… have you had a strong desire or urge to use (DRUG/MEDICATION) **in between those times when you were using** (DRUG/MEDICATION)?

    –   +   **C27**

C28

… have you missed work or school or often arrived late because you were intoxicated, high, or recovering from the night before?

How about …

…. doing a bad job at work or school, or failing courses, or getting kicked out of school because of your repeated use of (DRUG/MEDICATION)?

… getting into trouble at work or school because of your repeated use of (DRUG/MEDICATION)?

… not taking care of things at home because of your use of (DRUG/MEDICATION), **like paying bills, making sure food and clean clothes are available for your family, and making sure your children go to school and get medical care?**

    –   +   **C28**

C29	**During the past 12 months…** **… has your use of** (DRUG/MEDICATION) **caused problems with other people, such as with family members, friends, or people at work?** *IF YES*: **Did you keep on using** (DRUG/MEDICATION) **anyway?** *Note: Code "+" only if "YES" to both.*	– +	C29
C30	**… have you had to give up or reduce the time you spent at work, with family or friends, or on your hobbies because you were using** (DRUG/MEDICATION) **instead?**	– +	C30
C31	**… have you repeatedly gotten high before doing something that requires coordination and concentration like driving, boating, climbing on a ladder, or operating heavy machinery?** *IF YES*: **Would you say that your use of** (DRUG/MEDICATION) **affected your coordination or concentration so that it was more likely that you or someone else could have been hurt?** *Note: Code "+" only if "YES" to both.*	– +	C31
C32	**… has your use of** (DRUG/MEDICATION) **caused you any problems like making you very depressed, anxious, paranoid, very irritable, or extremely agitated?** **… has your use of** (DRUG/MEDICATION) **ever caused physical problems, like heart palpitations, coughing or trouble breathing, constipation, or skin infections?** *IF YES TO EITHER OF ABOVE*: **Did you keep on using** (DRUG/MEDICATION) **anyway?** *Note: Code "+" only if "YES" to both parts.*	– +	C32
C33	**… have you found that you needed to use much more** (DRUG/MEDICATION) **than when you first started using it to get the feeling you wanted or that when you used the same amount, it had much less effect than before?** *IF PRESCRIBED MEDICATION*: **Did you repeatedly take more of** (DRUG/MEDICATION) **than was prescribed, or run out of your prescription early?**	– +	C33

C34	**… have you ever had any withdrawal symptoms, like feeling sick when you cut down or stopped using** (DRUG/MEDICATION) **after a period of heavy or prolonged use of** (DRUG/MEDICATION)**?**
	
	    *IF YES: <u>Refer to the criteria for the appropriate substance-specific withdrawal syndrome on **page C-8** and rate item as "+" if full criteria have been met.</u>*
	
	After not using (DRUG/MEDICATION) **for a few hours or more, did you sometimes use it or something like it to keep yourself from getting sick with** (WITHDRAWAL SYMPTOMS)**?**
	
	    IF PRESCRIBED MEDICATION: **Were you taking this exactly as your doctor told you to? (Did you ever take more of it than was prescribed or run out of your prescription early? Did you ever have to go to more than one doctor to make sure you didn't run out?)**
		– +	C34

C35

*If at least <u>two</u> items (**C24–C34**) are coded "+":*

<u>Diagnose</u> **Nonalcohol Substance Use Disorder**, *indicating name of substance:* _____

___ *Mild Nonalcohol Substance Use Disorder (if 2–3 symptoms),*
___ *Moderate Nonalcohol Substance Use Disorder (if 4–5 symptoms), or*
___ *Severe Nonalcohol Substance Use Disorder (if 6 or more symptoms)*

*and then continue with **next module.***

*Otherwise, continue with **next module.***

C35

DSM-5 Criteria for Substance-Specific Withdrawal Syndromes

Listed below are the characteristic withdrawal syndromes for those classes of psychoactive substances for which a withdrawal syndrome has been identified. *(NOTE: A specific withdrawal syndrome has not been identified for PCP, HALLUCINOGENS, or INHALANTS.)* Withdrawal symptoms may occur following the cessation of prolonged moderate or heavy use of a psychoactive substance or a reduction in the amount used.

SEDATIVES, HYPNOTICS, OR ANXIOLYTICS

Two (or more) of the following, developing within several hours to a few days after the cessation of (or reduction in) sedative, hypnotic, or anxiolytic use that has been prolonged:

1. Autonomic hyperactivity (e.g., sweating or pulse rate greater than 100 bpm)
2. Hand tremor
3. Insomnia
4. Nausea or vomiting
5. Transient visual, tactile, or auditory hallucinations or illusions
6. Psychomotor agitation
7. Anxiety
8. Grand mal seizures

CANNABIS

Three (or more) of the following signs and symptoms developing within approximately 1 week after cessation of cannabis use that has been heavy and prolonged (i.e., usually daily or almost daily use over a period of at least a few months):

1. Irritability, anger, or aggression
2. Nervousness or anxiety
3. Sleep difficulty (e.g., insomnia, disturbing dreams)
4. Decreased appetite or weight loss
5. Restlessness
6. Depressed mood
7. At least one of the following physical symptoms causing significant discomfort: abdominal pain, shakiness/tremors, sweating, fever, chills, or headache

STIMULANTS/COCAINE

Dysphoric mood AND two (or more) of the following physiological changes, developing within a few hours to several days after cessation of (or reduction in) prolonged amphetamine-type substance, cocaine, or other stimulant use:

1. Fatigue
2. Vivid, unpleasant dreams
3. Insomnia or hypersomnia
4. Increased appetite
5. Psychomotor retardation or agitation

OPIOIDS

Three (or more) of the following, developing within minutes to several days after cessation of (or reduction in) opioid use that has been heavy and prolonged (i.e., several weeks or longer) or after administration of an opioid antagonist after a period of opioid use:

1. Dysphoric mood
2. Nausea or vomiting
3. Muscle aches
4. Lacrimation or rhinorrhea (runny nose)
5. Pupillary dilation, piloerection (goose bumps), or sweating
6. Diarrhea
7. Yawning
8. Fever
9. Insomnia

D. ANXIETY DISORDERS

CURRENT PANIC DISORDER

D1	In the past 6 months, since (6 MONTHS AGO), **have you had an intense rush of anxiety, or what someone might call a "panic attack," when you <u>suddenly</u> felt very frightened or anxious or suddenly developed a lot of physical symptoms?**	– + **D1**

↓ *Skip to **D17** (Current Agoraphobia), **page D-3**.*

D2	**Have you had at least two attacks like this that came out of the blue—that is, in situations where you didn't expect to be nervous or uncomfortable?**	– + **D2**

↓ *Skip to **D17** (Current Agoraphobia), **page D-3**.*

Now think of the worst attack that you have experienced during the past 6 months.

During that attack ...

D3	... **did your heart race, pound, or skip?**	– + **D3**
D4	... **did you sweat?**	– + **D4**
D5	... **did you tremble or shake?**	– + **D5**
D6	... **were you short of breath? (Have trouble catching your breath? Feel like you were being smothered?)**	– + **D6**
D7	... **did you feel as if you were choking?**	– + **D7**
D8	... **did you have chest pain or pressure?**	– + **D8**
D9	... **did you have nausea or upset stomach or the feeling that you were going to have diarrhea?**	– + **D9**
D10	... **did you feel dizzy, unsteady, or like you might pass out?**	– + **D10**
D11	... **did you have flushes, hot flashes, or chills?**	– + **D11**

D12	... did you have tingling or numbness in parts of your body?	−	+	D1
D13	... did you have the feeling that you were detached from your body or mind, that time was moving slowly, or that you were an outside observer of your own thoughts or movements? How about feeling that everything around you was unreal or that you were in a dream?	−	+	D1
D14	... were you afraid you were going crazy or might lose control?	−	+	D1
D15	... were you afraid that you were dying?	−	+	D1

*If fewer than <u>four</u> items (**D2–D15**) are coded "+," skip to **D17** (Current Agoraphobia), **page D-3**. Otherwise, continue with **D16**.*

D16	After any of these attacks, for at least a month, were you concerned that you might have another attack or worried that you would have a heart attack or worried that you would lose control or go crazy? After any of these attacks, for at least a month, did you do anything differently because of the attacks, like avoiding certain places or not going out alone or avoiding certain activities like exercise or always making sure you're near a bathroom or exit? *Note: Code "+" if "YES" to either question.*	− + *Continue with **D17** (Current Agora-phobia), **Page D-3**.*	D1

Diagnose: Current Panic Disorder.

*IF A CONCURRENT MEDICAL CONDITION OR SUBSTANCE/MEDICATION USE, SKIP TO **MODULE J** TO RULE OUT ANXIETY DISORDER DUE TO ANOTHER MEDICAL CONDITION AND/OR SUBSTANCE-INDUCED ANXIETY DISORDER AND THEN RETURN HERE.*

*Continue with **D17** (Current Agoraphobia), **Page D-3**.*

CURRENT AGORAPHOBIA (PAST 6 MONTHS)

D17 — In the past 6 months, since (6 MONTHS AGO), **have you been very anxious about or afraid of a number of different situations like going out of the house alone, being in crowds, going to stores, standing in lines, or traveling on buses or trains?**

—   +   **D17**

*Skip to **D23** (Current Social Anxiety Disorder), **Page D-4**.*

D18 — **Have you been avoiding these situations because you have been afraid that it might be hard for you to get out of these situations if you absolutely needed to … like if you suddenly developed a panic attack or something else happened to you that would be embarrassing like passing out, falling, losing control of your bladder or bowels, or vomiting?**

—   +   **D18**

*Skip to **D23** (Current Social Anxiety Disorder), **Page D-4**.*

D19 — **Do you almost always feel frightened or anxious when you are in one of the situations that you avoid?**

—   +   **D19**

*Skip to **D23** (Current Social Anxiety Disorder), **Page D-4**.*

D20 — **Have you gone out of your way to avoid these situations?**

    IF NO: **Have you been able to go into one of these situations only if you are with someone you know?**

        IF NO: **When you have had to be in one of these situations, have you felt intensely afraid or anxious?**

—   +   **D20**

*Skip to **D23** (Current Social Anxiety Disorder), **Page D-4**.*

D21 — **Has your fear or avoidance been present for most of the past 6 months?**

—   +   **D21**

*Skip to **D23** (Current Social Anxiety Disorder), **Page D-4**.*

D22 — **Has your fear or avoidance of these situations affected your life in important ways?**

Are you very bothered by the fact that you are afraid of these situations?

Note: Code "+" if "YES" to either question.

—   +   **D22**

*Continue with **D23** (Current Social Anxiety Disorder), **Page D-4**.*

<u>Diagnose:</u> **Current Agoraphobia.**
*Continue with **D23** (Current Social Anxiety Disorder), **Page D-4**.*

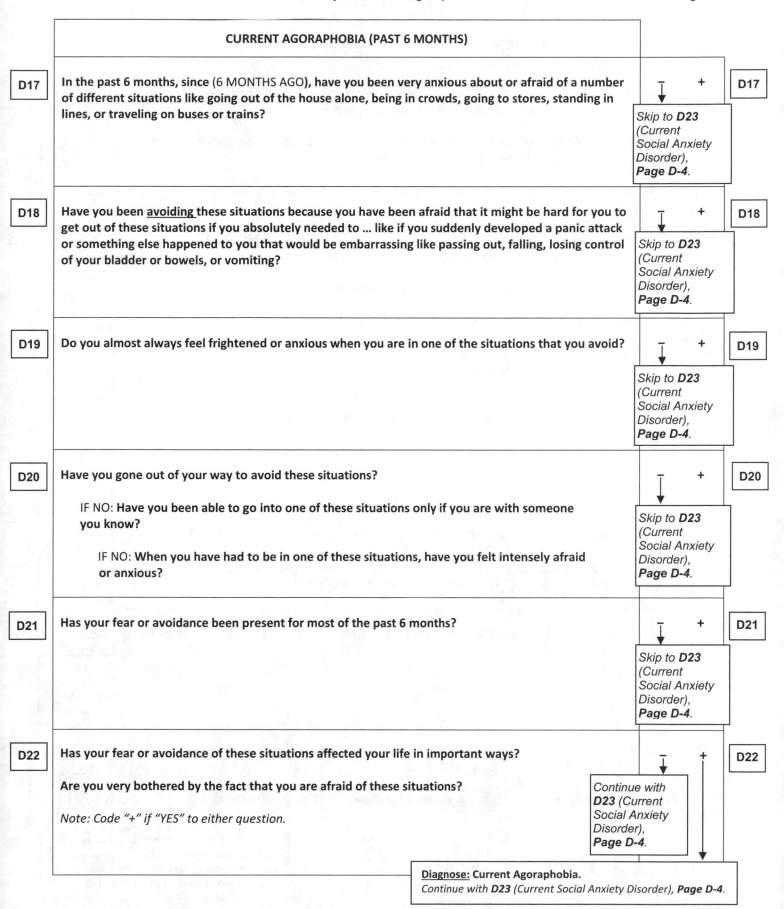

CURRENT SOCIAL ANXIETY DISORDER (PAST 6 MONTHS)

D23 | In the past 6 months, since (6 MONTHS AGO), **have you been especially nervous or anxious in social situations, like having a conversation or meeting unfamiliar people?**

Is there anything that you have been afraid to do or felt very uncomfortable doing in front of other people, like speaking, eating, writing, or using a public bathroom?

IF YES TO EITHER OF ABOVE: **Give me some examples of when this has happened.**

−   +

Skip to D29 (Current GAD), Page D-5.

D2

D24 | **Were you afraid of being embarrassed when you were in** (FEARED SOCIAL OR PERFORMANCE SITUATION[S]) **because of what you might say or how you might act?**

Were you afraid that this would lead to your being rejected by other people?

How about making others uncomfortable or offending them because of what you said or how you acted?

Note: Code "+" if "YES" to any of these questions.

−   +

Skip to D29 (Current GAD), Page D-5.

D2

D25 | **Have you almost always felt frightened when you were in** (FEARED SOCIAL OR PERFORMANCE SITUATION[S])**?**

−   +

Skip to D29 (Current GAD), Page D-5.

D2

D26 | **Have you gone out of your way to avoid** (FEARED SOCIAL OR PERFORMANCE SITUATION[S])**?**

If you were unable to avoid (FEARED SOCIAL OR PERFORMANCE SITUATION[S]) **was it very uncomfortable for you to be in** (FEARED SOCIAL OR PERFORMANCE SITUATION[S])**?**

−   +

Skip to D29 (Current GAD), Page D-5.

D2

D27 | **Has your fear or avoidance of** (FEARED SOCIAL OR PERFORMANCE SITUATION[S]) **been present for most of the past 6 months?**

−   +

Skip to D29 (Current GAD) Page D-5.

D2

D28 | **Has your fear or avoidance of** (FEARED SOCIAL OR PERFORMANCE SITUATION[S]) **affected your life in important ways?**

Are you very bothered by the fact that you are afraid of (FEARED SOCIAL OR PERFORMANCE SITUATION[S])**?**

−   +

Continue with D29 (Current GAD), Page D-5.

D2

<u>Diagnose:</u> **Current Social Anxiety Disorder.**
Continue with D29 (Current GAD), Page D-5.

CURRENT GENERALIZED ANXIETY DISORDER (PAST 6 MONTHS)

D29	Over the past 6 months, since (6 MONTHS AGO), **have you been feeling anxious and worried in general for more days than not?** *IF YES:* **Have you been worrying about a lot of different things, like your job, your health or your family members' health, your finances, or other less important things like being late for appointments, even when there was no real reason to worry?** *Note: Code "+" only if "YES" to both of the above questions.*	– ↓ + *Skip to next module.*	**D29**
D30	When worrying this way, **have you found that it's hard to stop yourself or to think about anything else?**	– ↓ + *Skip to next module.*	**D30**
D31	Thinking about those periods in the past 6 months when you were feeling nervous, anxious, or worried … **… have you often felt physically restless, like you couldn't sit still?** **… have you often felt keyed up or on edge?** *Note: Code "+" if "YES" to either question.*	– +	**D31**
D32	**… have you often tired easily?**	– +	**D32**
D33	**… have you often had trouble concentrating or has your mind often gone blank?**	– +	**D33**
D34	**… have you often been irritable?**	– +	**D34**
D35	**… have your muscles often been tense?**	– +	**D35**
D36	**… have you often had trouble falling or staying asleep? How about often feeling tired when you woke up because you didn't get a good night's sleep?**	– +	**D36**

*If fewer than <u>two</u> items **(D31–D36)** are coded "+," skip to **next module.** Otherwise, continue with **D37, page D-6.***

D37   **Have your anxiety and worry affected your life in important ways?**

Are you very bothered by the fact that you are anxious and worried most of the time?

D3

—   +

Skip to **next module**.

Diagnose: **Current Generalized Anxiety Disorder.**

*IF A CONCURRENT MEDICAL CONDITION OR SUBSTANCE/MEDICATION USE, SKIP TO **MODULE J** TO RULE OUT ANXIETY DISORDER DUE TO ANOTHER MEDICAL CONDITION AND/OR SUBSTANCE-INDUCED ANXIETY DISORDER AND THEN RETURN HERE.*

*Continue with **next module**.*

E. OBSESSIVE-COMPULSIVE DISORDER

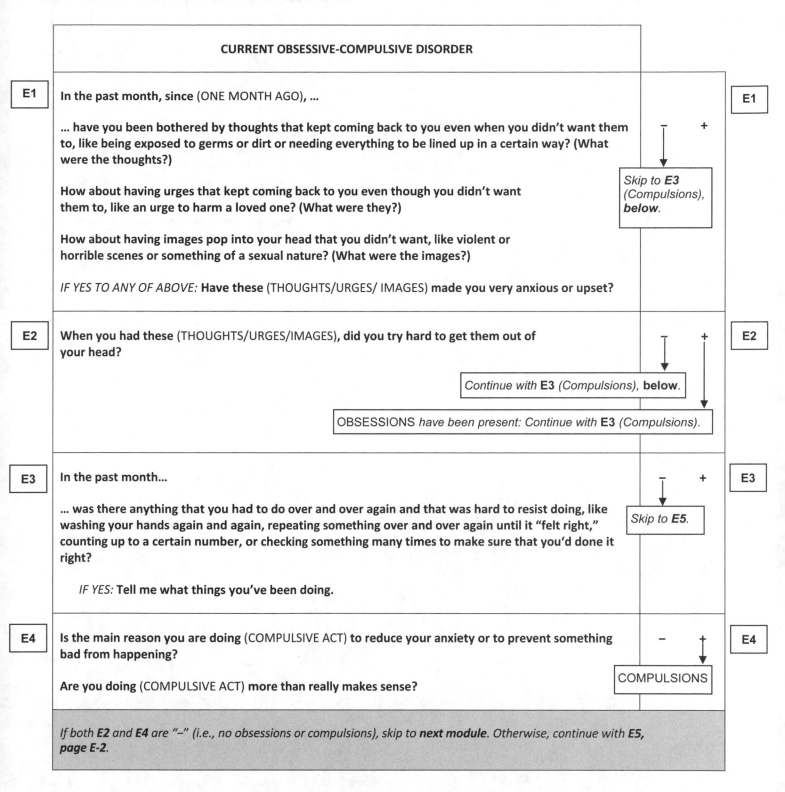

CURRENT OBSESSIVE-COMPULSIVE DISORDER

E1

In the past month, since (ONE MONTH AGO), ...

... **have you been bothered by thoughts that kept coming back to you even when you didn't want them to, like being exposed to germs or dirt or needing everything to be lined up in a certain way? (What were the thoughts?)**

How about having urges that kept coming back to you even though you didn't want them to, like an urge to harm a loved one? (What were they?)

How about having images pop into your head that you didn't want, like violent or horrible scenes or something of a sexual nature? (What were the images?)

IF YES TO ANY OF ABOVE: **Have these** (THOUGHTS/URGES/ IMAGES) **made you very anxious or upset?**

     −   +

Skip to E3 (Compulsions), below.

E1

E2

When you had these (THOUGHTS/URGES/IMAGES), **did you try hard to get them out of your head?**

     −   +

Continue with E3 (Compulsions), **below.**

OBSESSIONS *have been present: Continue with E3 (Compulsions).*

E2

E3

In the past month...

... **was there anything that you had to do over and over again and that was hard to resist doing, like washing your hands again and again, repeating something over and over again until it "felt right," counting up to a certain number, or checking something many times to make sure that you'd done it right?**

    IF YES: **Tell me what things you've been doing.**

     −   +

Skip to E5.

E3

E4

Is the main reason you are doing (COMPULSIVE ACT) **to reduce your anxiety or to prevent something bad from happening?**

Are you doing (COMPULSIVE ACT) **more than really makes sense?**

     −   +

COMPULSIONS

E4

If both E2 and E4 are "−" (i.e., no obsessions or compulsions), skip to next module. Otherwise, continue with E5, page E-2.

| E5 | **Have you spent at least an hour a day on** (OBSESSION or COMPULSION)?

Has (OBSESSION OR COMPULSION) **affected your life in important ways?**

Are you very bothered by the fact that you have (OBSESSION or COMPULSION)**?** | 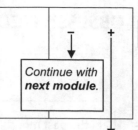 | E5 |

Continue with **next module**.

IF A CONCURRENT MEDICAL CONDITION OR SUBSTANCE/MEDICATION USE, SKIP TO **MODULE J** *TO RULE OUT OBSESSIVE-COMPULSIVE AND RELATED DISORDER DUE TO ANOTHER MEDICAL CONDITION AND/OR SUBSTANCE-INDUCED OBSESSIVE-COMPULSIVE AND RELATED DISORDER AND THEN RETURN HERE.*

<u>**Diagnose:**</u> **Current Obsessive-Compulsive Disorder.**
Continue with **next module**.

F. ADULT ATTENTION-DEFICIT/HYPERACTIVITY DISORDER

CURRENT ATTENTION-DEFICIT/HYPERACTIVITY DISORDER
(PAST 6 MONTHS, SUBJECTS/PATIENTS AGE 17 OR OLDER)

F1	Over the past several years, have you been easily distracted or disorganized? Over the past several years, have you had a lot of difficulty sitting still or waiting your turn?	− + *Skip to* ***next module***. **F1**
F2	Looking back over the past 6 months, since (6 MONTHS AGO), … … have you often missed important details or made mistakes at work (or school) or while taking care of things at home? … have you often made mistakes balancing your checkbook or paying bills? …. have other people often complained that you don't pay enough attention to detail or that your work is careless?	− + **F2**
F3	… have you often had trouble staying focused on things like reading a book, following a conversation, or doing household chores?	− + **F3**
F4	… have other people often commented or complained that you haven't seemed to be listening or that your mind was elsewhere while they were talking?	− + **F4**
F5	… have you often started things and then dropped them without finishing because you lost your focus or got sidetracked?	− + **F5**
F6	… have you often had trouble organizing things at home or at work or staying on top of things? … has your desk or closet often been so messy and disorganized that you have had trouble finding things? … have you often had trouble managing your time so that you have been late a lot or missed appointments or failed to meet deadlines?	− + **F6**

		–	+	
F7	Looking back over the past 6 months... ... have you typically avoided or strongly disliked tasks or jobs that require concentrating on details for extended periods, things like preparing a report for work or writing a paper?	–	+	**F7**
F8	... have you often lost or misplaced things like your wallet, your glasses, your keys, or your cell phone? How about files at work or tools you needed for work?	–	+	**F8**
F9	... have you often been very easily distracted by things going on around you that most others would have easily ignored, like a car honking or other people talking? Have you often gotten distracted by your own thoughts that were unrelated to what you were doing?	–	+	**F9**
F10	... have you often been very forgetful, for example, forgetting to return phone calls, forgetting to pay bills, or forgetting appointments?	–	+	**F10**
F11	*If more than <u>five</u> items (**F2–F10**) are coded "+," check here _____ (subject/patient has an <u>inattentive component</u> to the presentation). In all cases, continue with **F12**.*			**F11**
F12	Looking back over the past 6 months, since (6 MONTHS AGO), ... have you often fidgeted or squirmed or tapped your foot when you were in a situation where you have had to sit still, like on a plane, in class, or at meetings?	–	+	**F12**
F13	... have you often left your seat when you were expected to stay seated, for example, during a religious service, in a movie theater, in class, or at meetings?	–	+	**F13**
F14	... have you often felt physically restless, especially when you had to stay put for a while?	–	+	**F14**
F15	... have you often been unable to do something quietly in your free time, like reading a book? Have others complained that you are not able to do things quietly in your free time?	–	+	**F15**

		−	+	
F16	**Looking back over the past 6 months...**			**F16**
	... have you often felt like you always have to be moving or doing something?			
	... have you often been uncomfortable when you have to be still for some length of time?			
	... have others told you that you are hard to keep up with?			
	... have other people told you that being with you is exhausting or draining?			
F17	**... have you often talked too much?**	−	+	**F17**
	... have other people complained that you talk too much?			
F18	**...have you often finished people's sentences or blurted out an answer before the other person finished asking the question?**	−	+	**F18**
	... has it often been hard for you to wait your turn in conversations?			
F19	**... have you often had trouble waiting in line or ordering at a restaurant or waiting for your turn in other things?**	−	+	**F19**
F20	**... have you often interrupted other people while they were talking or barged into others' conversations?**	−	+	**F20**
	What about jumping in to take over what someone else was doing, like when someone is taking too long to unlock a door or fix something?			

F21	*If more than <u>five</u> items (**F12–F20**) are coded "+," check here _____ (subject/patient has a <u>hyperactive-impulsive component</u> to the presentation). In all cases, continue with **F22**.*	**F21**
	*If fewer than <u>five</u> of the inattentive items (**F2–F10**) are coded "+" (refer to item **F11**) AND fewer than <u>five</u> of the hyperactive-impulsive items (**F12–F20**) are coded "+" (refer to item **F21**), skip to **next module**. Otherwise, continue with **F22**.*	

F22   **Did you have any** (SXS RATED "+") **before you were 12?**

Did teachers complain that you were not paying attention or that you talked too much in class?

Were you ever sent to the principal's office because of your behavior?

Did your parents complain that you were not able to sit still, that you were very messy, or that you were never ready on time?

—   +

*Skip to **next module**.*

F23   **Have** (SXS RATED "+") **happened in more than one area of your life, like at school, at work, and at home?**

—   +

*Skip to **next module**.*

F24   **Have** (SXS RATED "+") **caused you any problems in your relationships with your family, romantic partners, or friends?**

Have they made it more difficult to do your work or schoolwork?

Have they affected the quality of your work or schoolwork?

Have they made it hard for you to do things that are important to you, like religious activities, physical exercise, sports, or hobbies?

Have (SXS RATED "+") affected any other important part of your life?

—   +

*Continue with **next module**.*

Diagnose: Current Attention-Deficit/Hyperactivity Disorder.
Specify type of presentation.

___ **Predominantly inattentive presentation** (if **F11** is checked and **F21** is not checked)
___ **Predominantly hyperactive-impulsive presentation** (if **F11** is not checked and **F21** is checked)
___ **Combined presentation** (if both **F11** and **F21** are checked)

*Continue with **next module**.*

G. POSTTRAUMATIC STRESS DISORDER

CURRENT POSTTRAUMATIC STRESS DISORDER

G1	I'd now like to ask about some things that may have happened to you over your lifetime that may have been extremely upsetting. Have you ever been in a life-threatening situation like a major disaster or fire, combat, or a serious car or work-related accident? What about being physically or sexually assaulted or abused or threatened with physical or sexual assault? How about seeing another person being physically or sexually assaulted or abused or threatened with physical or sexual assault? Have you ever seen another person killed or dead or badly hurt? How about learning that one of these things happened to someone you are close to?	– + **G1** ↓ *Skip to **next module**.*
G2	In the past month, since (ONE MONTH AGO), **have you had thoughts about** (ACKNOWLEDGED TRAUMATIC EVENT) **that kept coming back to you even when you don't want to think about it?** **How about bad dreams about** (TRAUMATIC EVENT) **or the feeling that you are back in the situation again?** **What about getting very upset or having physical symptoms—like breaking out in a sweat, or your heart pounding or racing, or feeling very upset when something or someone reminds you of** (TRAUMATIC EVENT)**?** *Note: Code "+" if "YES" to any of these questions.*	– + **G2** ↓ *Skip to **next module**.*
G3	In the past month, have you done things to avoid having thoughts and feelings similar to those you had during (TRAUMATIC EVENT), like keeping yourself busy, distracting yourself by playing computer or video games or watching TV, or using drugs or alcohol to "numb" yourself or try to forget what happened? Has this been for most of the time in the past month? *Note: Code "+" only if "YES" to both questions.*	– + **G3**
G4	In the past month, have there been specific things that you have tried to avoid because it could bring up upsetting memories, thoughts, or feelings about (TRAUMATIC EVENT)? Has this been most of the time during the past month? *Note: Code "+" only if "YES" to both questions.*	– + **G4**

*If both **G3** and **G4** are "–" (i.e., no avoidance), skip to **next module**. Otherwise, continue with **G5, next page**.*

G5	For most of the time during the past month, have you been unable to remember some important part of what happened? *IF YES:* **Did you get a head injury during (TRAUMATIC EVENT)? Were you drinking a lot or were you taking any drugs at the time of (TRAUMATIC EVENT)?** *Note: Code "+" only if answer to first question is "YES" and answer is "NO" to the follow-up question.*	– +	G
G6	For most of the time during the past month, has there been a change in how you thought about yourself compared with before (TRAUMATIC EVENT), **like feeling you were "bad" or permanently damaged or "broken"?** For most of the time during the past month, has there been a change in how you see other people or the way the world works compared with before (TRAUMATIC EVENT), **like feeling you can't trust anyone anymore or like the world is a completely dangerous place?**	– +	G
G7	For most of the past month, have you unreasonably blamed yourself for the (TRAUMATIC EVENT) **or how it affected your life, like thinking that** (TRAUMATIC EVENT) **was your fault or that you could have done something to prevent it or that you should have gotten over it by now?**	– +	G
G8	For most of the past month, have you had bad feelings a lot of the time, like feeling sad, angry, afraid, guilty, ashamed, or numb?	– +	G
G9	During most of the past month, have you been a lot less interested in things that you were interested in before (TRAUMATIC EVENT), **like spending time with family or friends, reading books, watching TV, cooking, or sports?**	– +	G
G10	For most of the past month, have you felt distant or disconnected from others or have you closed yourself off from other people?	– +	G
G11	For most of the past month, have you been unable to experience good feelings, like feeling happy, joyful, satisfied, loving, or tender toward other people?	– +	G
	*If fewer than <u>two</u> of the negative alterations in cognitions and mood associated with the traumatic event (**G5–G11**) are coded "+," skip to **next module**. Otherwise, continue with **G12, below**.*		
G12	In the past month, since (ONE MONTH AGO), **have you lost control of your anger over something little and threatened or hurt someone or damaged something?** In the past month, have you been more quick-tempered or had a shorter "fuse" than before?	– +	G

G13	In the past month, have you done reckless things, like driving dangerously or drinking or using drugs without caring about the consequences? **How about hurting yourself on purpose or trying to kill yourself? (What did you do?)**	–	+	G13
G14	In the past month, have you been more watchful or on guard or extra aware of your surroundings compared with how you were before (TRAUMATIC EVENT)?	–	+	G14
G15	In the past month, have you been jumpy or easily startled, like by sudden noises?	–	+	G15
G16	In the past month, have you had trouble concentrating?	–	+	G16
G17	In the past month, have you had difficulty falling asleep or staying asleep or had restless sleep?	–	+	G17

*If fewer than <u>two</u> of the marked alterations in arousal and reactivity associated with the traumatic event (**G12–G17**) are coded "+," skip to **next module**. Otherwise, continue with **G18, below**.*

G18	**Have your symptoms affected your life in important ways?** *IF NO:* **Are you very bothered by the fact that you have these symptoms?**	–	+	G18

Continue with **next module**.

Diagnose: Posttraumatic Stress Disorder (current).
*Continue with **next module**.*

H. EATING DISORDERS

CURRENT ANOREXIA NERVOSA

H1   **Have you had a time in the past 3 months, since** (THREE MONTHS AGO), **when you weighed much less than other people thought you ought to weigh?**

     IF YES: **What was your lowest weight in the past 3 months? How tall are you?**

*Note: Code "+" if weight is below the value in the table (in pounds or kilograms) given the person's height, which corresponds to a BMI of **17.0 kg/m²** (considered by WHO to indicate moderate or severe thinness):*

ft/in	4'9"	4'10"	4'11"	5'0"	5'1"	5'2"	5'3"	5'4"	5'5"	5'6"
lb	79	82	84	87	90	93	96	99	102	106
cm	145	147	150	152	155	158	160	163	165	168
kg	36	37	38.5	39.5	41	42.5	43.5	45.5	46.5	48

ft/in	5'7"	5'8"	5'9"	5'10"	5'11"	6'0"	6'1"	6'2"	6'3"	6'4"
lb	109	112	115	119	122	125	129	133	136	139
cm	170	173	175	178	180	183	185	188	191	194
kg	49	51	52	54	55	57	58.5	60	62	64

–   +

*Skip to **H4** (Current Bulimia Nervosa), **page H-2**.*

H2   **At that time, were you very afraid that you could become fat?**

Did you avoid high-calorie foods or high-fat foods or did you purposely throw up after you had eaten or do something else like take laxatives or diuretics, or exercise vigorously, to keep from gaining any weight?

–   +

*Skip to **H4** (Current Bulimia Nervosa), **page H-2**.*

H3   **At your lowest weight, did you still feel too fat or that part of your body was too fat?**

Did you need to be very thin in order to feel better about yourself?

–   +

*Continue with **H4** (Current Bulimia Nervosa), **page H-2**.*

Diagnose: Current Anorexia Nervosa. *Skip to **next module**.*

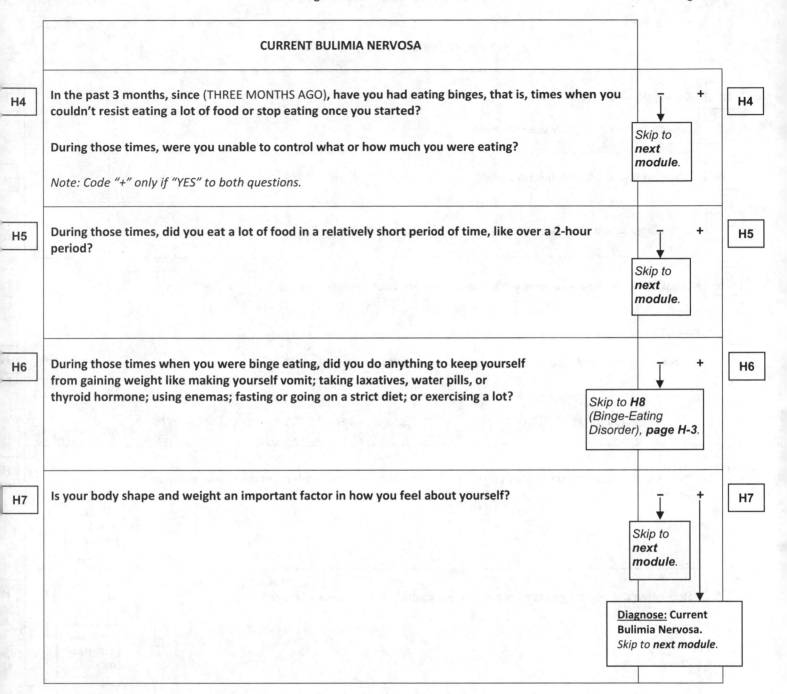

CURRENT BULIMIA NERVOSA

H4

In the past 3 months, since (THREE MONTHS AGO), **have you had eating binges, that is, times when you couldn't resist eating a lot of food or stop eating once you started?**

During those times, were you unable to control what or how much you were eating?

Note: Code "+" only if "YES" to both questions.

– +

↓

*Skip to **next module**.*

H4

H5

During those times, did you eat a lot of food in a relatively short period of time, like over a 2-hour period?

– +

↓

*Skip to **next module**.*

H5

H6

During those times when you were binge eating, did you do anything to keep yourself from gaining weight like making yourself vomit; taking laxatives, water pills, or thyroid hormone; using enemas; fasting or going on a strict diet; or exercising a lot?

– +

↓

*Skip to **H8** (Binge-Eating Disorder), **page H-3**.*

H6

H7

Is your body shape and weight an important factor in how you feel about yourself?

– +

↓

*Skip to **next module**.*

Diagnose: Current Bulimia Nervosa.
*Skip to **next module**.*

H7

CURRENT BINGE-EATING DISORDER

H8	During these binges did you... ... eat much more rapidly than normal?	– +	H
H9	... eat until you felt uncomfortably full?	– +	H
H10	... eat large amounts of food when you didn't feel physically hungry?	– +	H
H11	... eat alone because you were embarrassed by how much you were eating?	– +	H
H12	... feel disgusted with yourself, depressed, or very guilty after overeating?	– +	H

If fewer than three items (H8–H12) are coded "+," skip to next module. Otherwise, continue with H13.

H13	Was it very upsetting to you that you couldn't stop eating or control what or how much you were eating?	↓ + *Skip to* **next module**.	H
H14	How often did you binge eat over the past 3 months? At least once a week?	– + ↓ ↓ *Continue with* **next module**. **Diagnose:** Current Binge-Eating Disorder. *Continue with* **next module**.	H

I. SCREENING FOR OTHER DISORDERS

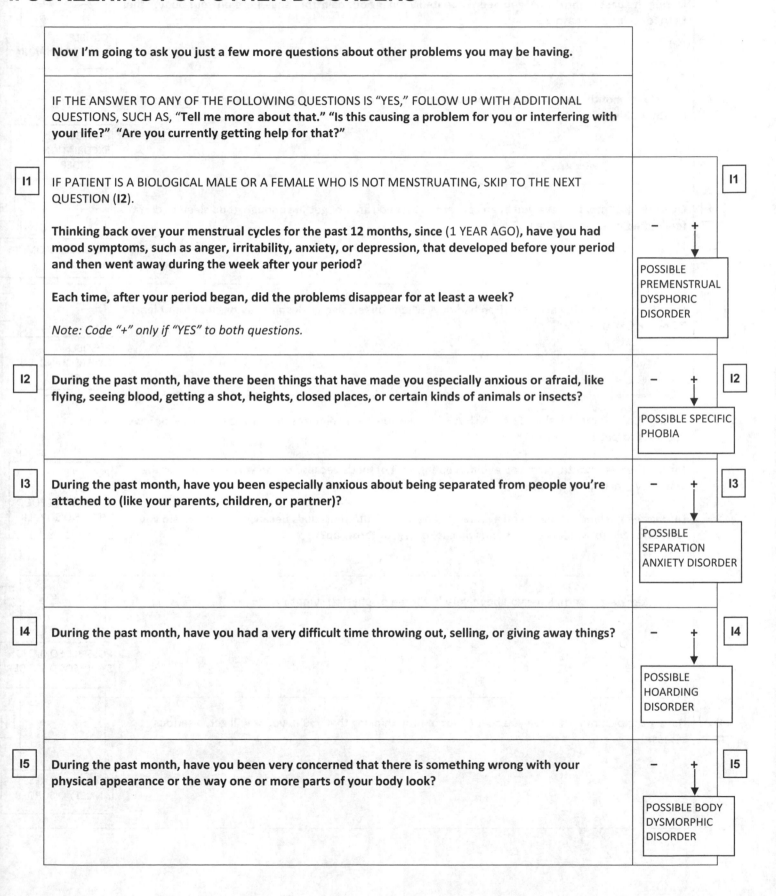

Now I'm going to ask you just a few more questions about other problems you may be having.

IF THE ANSWER TO ANY OF THE FOLLOWING QUESTIONS IS "YES," FOLLOW UP WITH ADDITIONAL QUESTIONS, SUCH AS, **"Tell me more about that." "Is this causing a problem for you or interfering with your life?" "Are you currently getting help for that?"**

I1

IF PATIENT IS A BIOLOGICAL MALE OR A FEMALE WHO IS NOT MENSTRUATING, SKIP TO THE NEXT QUESTION (**I2**).

Thinking back over your menstrual cycles for the past 12 months, since (1 YEAR AGO), have you had mood symptoms, such as anger, irritability, anxiety, or depression, that developed before your period and then went away during the week after your period?

Each time, after your period began, did the problems disappear for at least a week?

Note: Code "+" only if "YES" to both questions.

   −   +   **I1**

POSSIBLE PREMENSTRUAL DYSPHORIC DISORDER

I2   **During the past month, have there been things that have made you especially anxious or afraid, like flying, seeing blood, getting a shot, heights, closed places, or certain kinds of animals or insects?**

   −   +   **I2**

POSSIBLE SPECIFIC PHOBIA

I3   **During the past month, have you been especially anxious about being separated from people you're attached to (like your parents, children, or partner)?**

   −   +   **I3**

POSSIBLE SEPARATION ANXIETY DISORDER

I4   **During the past month, have you had a very difficult time throwing out, selling, or giving away things?**

   −   +   **I4**

POSSIBLE HOARDING DISORDER

I5   **During the past month, have you been very concerned that there is something wrong with your physical appearance or the way one or more parts of your body look?**

   −   +   **I5**

POSSIBLE BODY DYSMORPHIC DISORDER

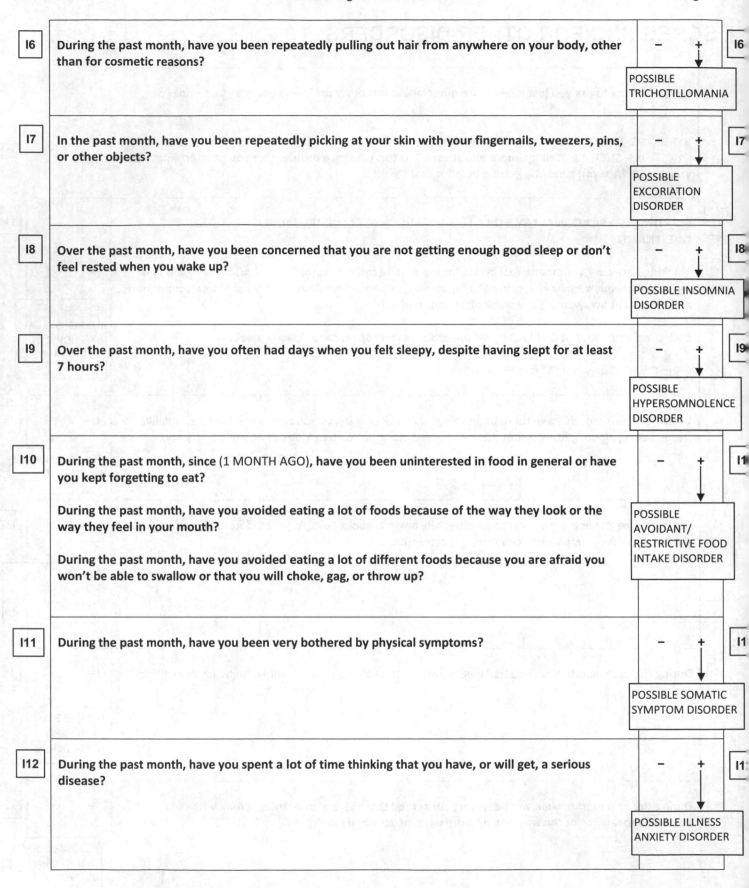

I6   During the past month, have you been repeatedly pulling out hair from anywhere on your body, other than for cosmetic reasons?   −   +   **I6**

POSSIBLE TRICHOTILLOMANIA

I7   In the past month, have you been repeatedly picking at your skin with your fingernails, tweezers, pins, or other objects?   −   +   **I7**

POSSIBLE EXCORIATION DISORDER

I8   Over the past month, have you been concerned that you are not getting enough good sleep or don't feel rested when you wake up?   −   +   **I8**

POSSIBLE INSOMNIA DISORDER

I9   Over the past month, have you often had days when you felt sleepy, despite having slept for at least 7 hours?   −   +   **I9**

POSSIBLE HYPERSOMNOLENCE DISORDER

I10   During the past month, since (1 MONTH AGO), have you been uninterested in food in general or have you kept forgetting to eat?   −   +   **I1**

During the past month, have you avoided eating a lot of foods because of the way they look or the way they feel in your mouth?

During the past month, have you avoided eating a lot of different foods because you are afraid you won't be able to swallow or that you will choke, gag, or throw up?

POSSIBLE AVOIDANT/ RESTRICTIVE FOOD INTAKE DISORDER

I11   During the past month, have you been very bothered by physical symptoms?   −   +   **I1**

POSSIBLE SOMATIC SYMPTOM DISORDER

I12   During the past month, have you spent a lot of time thinking that you have, or will get, a serious disease?   −   +   **I1**

POSSIBLE ILLNESS ANXIETY DISORDER

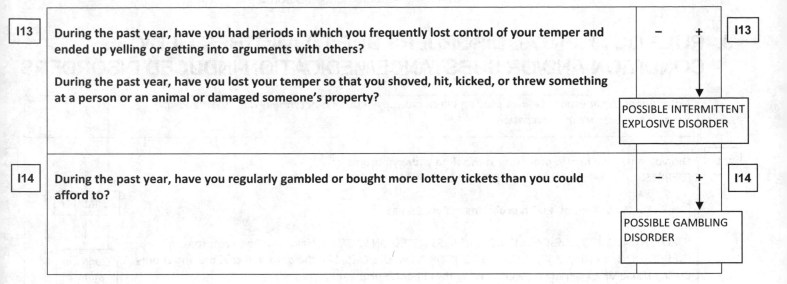

I13   During the past year, have you had periods in which you frequently lost control of your temper and ended up yelling or getting into arguments with others?

During the past year, have you lost your temper so that you shoved, hit, kicked, or threw something at a person or an animal or damaged someone's property?

−   +   **I13**

POSSIBLE INTERMITTENT EXPLOSIVE DISORDER

I14   During the past year, have you regularly gambled or bought more lottery tickets than you could afford to?

−   +   **I14**

POSSIBLE GAMBLING DISORDER

J. RULE OUT MENTAL DISORDERS DUE TO ANOTHER MEDICAL CONDITION AND/OR SUBSTANCE/MEDICATION-INDUCED DISORDERS

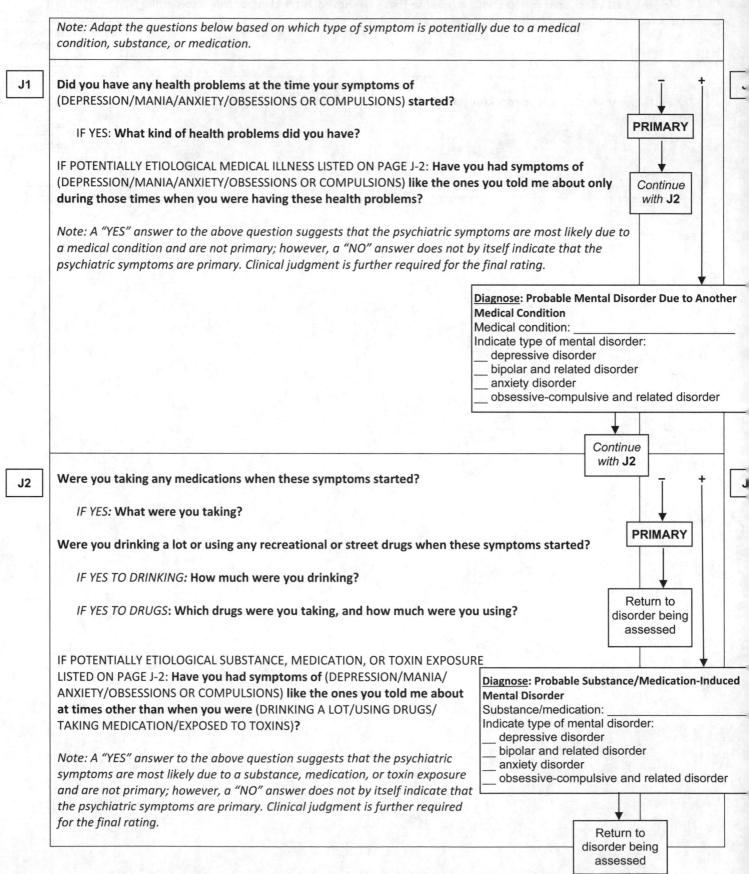

Note: Adapt the questions below based on which type of symptom is potentially due to a medical condition, substance, or medication.

J1

Did you have any health problems at the time your symptoms of (DEPRESSION/MANIA/ANXIETY/OBSESSIONS OR COMPULSIONS) **started?**

IF YES: **What kind of health problems did you have?**

IF POTENTIALLY ETIOLOGICAL MEDICAL ILLNESS LISTED ON PAGE J-2: **Have you had symptoms of** (DEPRESSION/MANIA/ANXIETY/OBSESSIONS OR COMPULSIONS) **like the ones you told me about only during those times when you were having these health problems?**

Note: A "YES" answer to the above question suggests that the psychiatric symptoms are most likely due to a medical condition and are not primary; however, a "NO" answer does not by itself indicate that the psychiatric symptoms are primary. Clinical judgment is further required for the final rating.

– +

PRIMARY

Continue with J2

Diagnose: Probable Mental Disorder Due to Another Medical Condition
Medical condition: _____
Indicate type of mental disorder:
__ depressive disorder
__ bipolar and related disorder
__ anxiety disorder
__ obsessive-compulsive and related disorder

Continue with J2

J2

Were you taking any medications when these symptoms started?

IF YES: **What were you taking?**

Were you drinking a lot or using any recreational or street drugs when these symptoms started?

IF YES TO DRINKING: **How much were you drinking?**

IF YES TO DRUGS: **Which drugs were you taking, and how much were you using?**

IF POTENTIALLY ETIOLOGICAL SUBSTANCE, MEDICATION, OR TOXIN EXPOSURE LISTED ON PAGE J-2: **Have you had symptoms of** (DEPRESSION/MANIA/ANXIETY/OBSESSIONS OR COMPULSIONS) **like the ones you told me about at times other than when you were** (DRINKING A LOT/USING DRUGS/TAKING MEDICATION/EXPOSED TO TOXINS)**?**

Note: A "YES" answer to the above question suggests that the psychiatric symptoms are most likely due to a substance, medication, or toxin exposure and are not primary; however, a "NO" answer does not by itself indicate that the psychiatric symptoms are primary. Clinical judgment is further required for the final rating.

– +

PRIMARY

Return to disorder being assessed

Diagnose: Probable Substance/Medication-Induced Mental Disorder
Substance/medication: _____
Indicate type of mental disorder:
__ depressive disorder
__ bipolar and related disorder
__ anxiety disorder
__ obsessive-compulsive and related disorder

Return to disorder being assessed

CAUSES OF DEPRESSIVE SYMPTOMS

Medical conditions known to cause depression include stroke, Huntington's disease, Parkinson's disease, traumatic brain injury, Cushing's disease, hypothyroidism, multiple sclerosis, and systemic lupus erythematosus.

Substances known to cause depression include alcohol (I/W); phencyclidine (I); hallucinogens (I); inhalants (I); opioids (I/W); sedatives, hypnotics, or anxiolytics (I/W); amphetamine and other stimulants (I/W); and cocaine (I/W).

Medications known to cause depression include antiviral agents (efavirenz); cardiovascular agents (clonidine, guanethidine, methyldopa, reserpine); retinoic acid derivatives (isotretinoin); antidepressants; anticonvulsants; anti-migraine agents (triptans); antipsychotics; hormonal agents (corticosteroids, oral contraceptives, gonadotropin-releasing hormone agonists, tamoxifen); smoking cessation agents (varenicline); and immunological agents (interferon).

CAUSES OF MANIC SYMPTOMS

Medical conditions known to cause mania include Alzheimer's disease, vascular dementia, HIV-induced dementia, Huntington's disease, Lewy body disease, Wernicke-Korsakoff syndrome, Cushing's disease, multiple sclerosis, amyotrophic lateral sclerosis, Parkinson's disease, Pick's disease, Creutzfeldt-Jakob disease, stroke, traumatic brain injuries, and hyperthyroidism.

Substances known to cause mania include alcohol (I/W); phencyclidine (I); hallucinogens (I); sedatives, hypnotics, and anxiolytics (I/W); amphetamines (I/W); and cocaine (I/W).

Medications known to cause mania include corticosteroids, androgens, isoniazid, levodopa, interferon-alpha, varenicline, procarbazine, clarithromycin, and ciprofloxacin.

CAUSES OF PANIC ATTACKS AND SYMPTOMS OF ANXIETY

Medical conditions known to cause panic attacks or anxiety include endocrine disease (e.g., hyperthyroidism, pheochromocytoma, hypoglycemia, hyperadrenocorticism), cardiovascular disorders (e.g., congestive heart failure, pulmonary embolism, arrhythmia such as atrial fibrillation), respiratory illness (e.g., chronic obstructive pulmonary disease, asthma, pneumonia), metabolic disturbances (e.g., vitamin B_{12} deficiency, porphyria), and neurological illness (e.g., neoplasms, vestibular dysfunction, encephalitis, seizure disorders).

Substances known to cause panic attacks or anxiety include alcohol (I/W); caffeine (I); cannabis (I); opioids (W); phencyclidine (I); other hallucinogens (I); inhalants (I); stimulants (including cocaine) (I/W); sedatives, hypnotics, and anxiolytics (W).

Medications known to cause panic attacks or anxiety include anesthetics and analgesics; sympathomimetics or other bronchodilators; anticholinergics; insulin; thyroid preparations; oral contraceptives; antihistamines; antiparkinsonian medications; corticosteroids; antihypertensive and cardiovascular medications; anticonvulsants; lithium carbonate; antipsychotic medications; antidepressant medications.

Toxins known to cause panic attacks or anxiety include heavy metals, organophosphate insecticides, nerve gases, carbon monoxide, carbon dioxide, and volatile substances such as gasoline and paint.

CAUSES OF OBSESSIONS AND COMPULSIONS

Medical conditions known to cause obsessions or compulsions include Sydenham's chorea and medical conditions leading to striatal damage, such as cerebral infarction.

Substances known to cause obsessions or compulsions include intoxication with cocaine, amphetamines, or other stimulants and exposure to heavy metals.